Drug and Alcohol Abuse

A Clinical Guide to Diagnosis and Treatment

CRITICAL ISSUES IN PSYCHIATRY
An Educational Series for Residents and Clinicians

Series Editor: **Sherwyn M. Woods, M.D., Ph.D.**
University of Southern California School of Medicine
Los Angeles, California

A RESIDENT'S GUIDE TO PSYCHIATRIC EDUCATION
Edited by Michael G. G. Thompson, M.D.

STATES OF MIND: Analysis of Change in Psychotherapy
Mardi J. Horowitz, M.D.

DRUG AND ALCOHOL ABUSE: A Clinical Guide to
Diagnosis and Treatment
Marc A. Schuckit, M.D.

**THE INTERFACE BETWEEN THE PSYCHODYNAMIC AND
BEHAVIORAL THERAPIES**
Edited by Judd Marmor, M.D. and Sherwyn M. Woods, M.D., Ph.D.

A Continuation Order Plan is available for this series. A continuation order will bring delivery of each new volume immediately upon publication. Volumes are billed only upon actual shipment. For further information please contact the publisher.

Drug and Alcohol Abuse

A Clinical Guide to Diagnosis and Treatment

Marc A. Schuckit, M.D.

San Diego Veterans Administration Medical Center
and
University of California, San Diego
School of Medicine

Plenum Medical Book Company · New York and London

Library of Congress Cataloging in Publicaton Data

Schuckit, Marc A
  Drug and alcohol abuse.

  (Critical issues in psychiatry)
  Includes bibliographical references and index.
  1. Drug abuse. 2 Alcoholism. I. Title. II. Series: [DNLM: 1. Alcoholism.
2. Drug abuse—Diagnosis. 3. Drug abuse—Therapy. WM270.3S384d]
RC566.S29   616.8'6   78-27854
ISBN 0-306-40215-7

First Printing — August 1979
Second Printing — September 1981

©1979 Plenum Publishing Corporation
233 Spring Street, New York, N.Y. 10013

Plenum Medical Book Company is an imprint of Plenum Publishing Corporation

Printed in the United States of America

To Sam who taught me how to laugh,
Lil who showed me how to love those close to me,
and to Judy, Dena, and Jordan who keep me doing both.

Foreword

When this series was conceived, a book on substance abuse, including alcohol and alcoholism, was to be of highest priority. This priority was a reflection of my view that the subject is often taught inadequately or insufficiently in many training programs. Yet these problems are commonly encountered in clinical practice, and all too often in situations where accurate diagnosis and rapid treatment are of critical importance. We wanted a book that would be concise and easily readable but also comprehensive in its presentation of the basic principles underlying clinical manifestations, diagnosis, and management. It was of particular importance that the book also serve as an easy reference guide in emergency situations.

Marc Schuckit, a man with impeccable credentials as a scholar and an experienced clinician in this field, has produced just such a book! Few psychiatrists, psychotherapists, or physicians will want to be without it. The presentation is comprehensive and in depth, yet so clear and well organized that it will also likely be of interest to medical students, nurses, and emergency personnel.

There are chapters on CNS depressants; alcohol and alcoholism; stimulants; opiates and other analgesics; cannabinols; hallucinogens; glues, solvents, and aerosols; and over-the-counter drugs. There are also chapters on multidrug use, on rehabilitation, and a rapid guide to emergency problems. Whether one's goal is an understanding of each drug class and its associated clinical problems or the need to diagnose rapidly and treat a specific drug emergency, the reader is led step by step through all the elements underlying the mechanism of action, the clinical and laboratory findings, and the specifics of treatment.

Since substance abuse is such a complicated and pervasive problem, and one that has resisted our attempts at primary prevention, this topic will continue to be of critical importance in clinical practice.

SHERWYN M. WOODS, M.D., PH.D.
Series Editor

Preface

This book grew out of a series of lectures developed to help the non-pharmacologist make sense out of a complex literature. The core of my approach is to learn the characteristics of drug classes, understand the usual types of difficulties associated with drugs, and then apply these general rules in clinical settings. It is hoped that the text will be a beginning place for gathering knowledge about drug types in the classroom and also a first step in handling emergency problems in clinical setting.

So that the book may properly serve as a resource for survey courses and as an emergency handbook, I have kept my comments relatively short, attempting to relate the most essential material. In order to help the reader understand drugs of abuse in greater depth, each chapter is highly referenced in the hopes that he will further expand his knowledge in this area.

I have never read a perfect manuscript or book, and (the views of my mother aside) this is not one. As with any complex endeavor, a series of compromises must be made as one decides whether to pursue Road A or Road B. My aim is to have this text strike a proper balance between the immediate needs of the clinician and those of the student looking for an introduction to substances of abuse.

I wish to extend my appreciation to Jane Ramsey, Edna Glenn, and my colleagues at the Alcoholism and Drug Abuse Institute of the University of Washington, as well as to my wife, Judy, and my colleagues at the University of California at San Diego Medical School, Department of Psychiatry, for their help in preparing this manuscript.

Marc A. Schuckit, M.D.

Contents

CHAPTER 1

An Overview

1.1. INTRODUCTION

This book is written for the medical student, the physician in practice, the psychologist, the social worker, and other health professionals, or paraprofessionals who need a quick, handy, clinically oriented reference on alcohol abuse and other drug problems. The first chapter addresses the need to learn the drug classes and the relevant problem areas from which generalizations can be made.

The book is divided into consecutive chapters dealing with specific classes of drugs. The discussion within each chapter is subdivided into sections on general information on the drugs in that class and sections covering the problems faced in emergency situations. Material on rehabiliation is presented in Chapter 13.

The text can be used in at least two basic ways:

1. If you are treating an emergency problem and know the probable class of the drug involved, you will turn to the emergency problem section of the relevant chapter. If you don't know the drug and need some general emergency guidelines, you will use the appropriate subsections of Chapters 1 and 12. Emphasis is placed on the most relevant drug-related material, and it is assumed that the reader already has some working knowledge of physical diagnosis, laboratory procedures, and the treatment of life-threatening emergencies.

Once the emergency has been handled, you will want to review the general information available on that class of drugs. At your leisure, you might then review the general information presented in Chapter 1 and go on to read the first section and some of the references cited in the bibliography of the relevant chapter.

2. If you are interested in learning about drug classes and their possible emergency problems, you should begin by skimming all the

1

chapters. After gaining some level of comfort with the general thrust of the material, you can then reread in detail those sections of most interest to you, going on to the more pertinent references. The first section of each chapter contains as little medical jargon as possible.

To address these goals and to make each chapter as self-sufficient as possible (in the emergency room you don't want to have to jump too much from chapter to chapter), there is some level of redundancy between book sections. I have tried, however, to strike a balance between readability and clinical usefulness.

No short handbook can answer all questions about every drug. The emergency-oriented nature of this text also tends to lead to oversimplification of rather complex problems. While you won't know everything about drugs after finishing the text, it is a place to start learning.

In order to present the material in the most efficient way, a number of shortcuts have been used. First, in giving the generic names of medications, I have deleted the suffix indicating which salt form is used (e.g., *chlordiazepoxide hydrochloride* is noted as *chlordiazepoxide*) because to list them would add little useful information. Secondly, the specific medications recommended for treatment in the emergency room settings represent the idiosyncrasies of my personal experience as well as those of other authors in the literature. The physician will usually be able to substitute another drug of the same class so that he can use a medication with which he has had experience (for example, when I note the use of haloperidol [Haldol], the physician might substitute *comparable* doses of trifluoperazine [Stelazine]). Thirdly, the dose ranges listed for the medications recommended for treatment of emergency situations are *approximations only* and will have to be modified for the individual patient based on the clinical setting and the patient's characteristics. Fourthly, although treatment discussions are frequently offered as a series of steps (as seen in most discussions of toxic reactions), the order offered is a general guideline that is to be modified for the particular clinical setting. Finally, it must be noted that the appropriate place for treating most emergency problems recorded here is in a hospital.

I have attempted to utilize the limited amount of space I have in a manner that reflects the frequency with which the usual clinician encounters drug problems. Therefore, the greatest amount of material is presented for the most clinically important drug, alcohol. Also, alcohol and opiates, drugs on which the most data for rehabilitation are available, are used as prototypes for the other discussions of rehabilitation.

Two final notes which reflect the sensitivities of our times are needed. To save time and space, male pronouns are consistently used in the text but are meant to refer to both genders. For similar goals of efficiency, the terms client, patient, and subject are used interchangeably.

1.2. SOME DEFINITIONS

Before we can begin, it is important to set forth a series of clinical concepts central to the discussion of substance misuse. The definitions presented are not the most pharmacologically sophisticated but do, I think, represent the greatest potential for use in clinical situations. To arrive at these terms, I have borrowed from a wide variety of standard texts and published studies attempting to blend them together into a readily utilizable framework.

1.2.1. Drug of Abuse

A *drug of abuse* is any substance, taken through any route of administration, that alters the mood, the level of perception, or brain functioning.[1] Such drugs include substances ranging from prescribed medications to alcohol to solvents.[2,3] All these substances are capable of producing changes in mood and altered states of learning.

1.2.2. Drug Abuse

Drug Abuse is the use of a mind-altering substance in a way that differs from generally approved medical or social practices.[4] Said in another way, when the continued use of a mind-altering substance means more to the individual than the problems caused by such use, the individual can be said to be abusing drugs.

1.2.3. Dependence

Dependence, also called habituation or compulsive use,[4] connotes a psychological and/or physical "need" for the drug.[1,4]

1. *Psychological dependence* is an attribute of all drugs of abuse[1] and centers on the user's needing the drug in order to reach a maximum level of functioning or feeling of well-being. This is a subjective term that is almost impossible to quantify, and thus it is of limited usefulness.

2. *Physical dependence* indicates the body's physiologic adaptation to chronic use of the substance, with the development of symptoms when the drug is stopped or withdrawn. While initially this concept appears quite simple, there is evidence that behavioral conditioning and psychological factors are important in what is usually felt to be a physical withdrawal syndrome.[5,6] There are two important aspects to physical dependence:

  a. *Tolerance* is the toleration of higher and higher doses of the drug or, said another way, the need for higher and higher doses to achieve the same effects. The phenomenon occurs both through alterations in drug metabolism, where the liver destroys the substance more quickly *(metabolic tolerance)*, and through alterations in the target cells' (usually in the nervous system) functioning in the presence of the drug, where tissue reaction to the drug is diminished *(pharmacodynamic tolerance)*. This is not an all-or-none phenomenon, and an individual may develop tolerance to one aspect of a drug's action and not another. The development of tolerance to one drug of a class usually indicates *cross-tolerance* to other drugs of the same class.[4]

b. *Withdrawal* is the appearance of physiologic symptoms when the drug is stopped too quickly. This phenomenon was first and most completely described for drugs like opiates or drugs that tend to depress the action of the central nervous system. However, there is evidence for withdrawal signs when drugs with different actions, such as stimulants, are used. As with tolerance, withdrawal is not an all-or-none phenomenon and usually consists of a syndrome of mixtures of a wide variety of possible symptoms.[4]

1.3. GENERAL COMMENTS ABOUT DRUG MECHANISMS

The drugs discussed here all affect the brain or the central nervous system (CNS). Unfortunately for our simplistic discussion, the actions of these drugs on the CNS tend to be highly complex. These factors are mediated through different neurotransmitters acting through a myriad of intercellular communications that strike a balance between excitatory and inhibitory functions.[7] This highly complex level of interaction, along with the drive of the nervous system to achieve equilibrium or homeostasis, makes it very difficult to generalize about specific mechanisms of drug actions.

The problems of understanding what to expect with a specific drug are even more complex for drugs bought "on the street." Most of these substances are not pure, and many (almost 100% for such drugs as THC; see Section 1.4.4.) do not even contain the purported major substances. Thus, one must apply the general lessons discussed in this text carefully, staying alert for unexpected consequences when treating drug abusers.

1.4. ONE APPROACH TO DRUG CLASSIFICATION

It is possible to learn the characteristics of a drug class and then to apply the general rules to the specific case. There are many possible

Table 1.1
Drug Classification Used in This Text

Class	Some examples
(General CNS) depressants	Alcohol, hypnotics, antianxiety drugs
CNS sympathomimetic or stimulants	Amphetamine, methylphenidate, cocaine, weight-loss products
Opiates	Heroin, morphine, methadone, propoxyphene
Cannabinols	Marijuana, hashish
Psychedelics or hallucinogens	LSD, mescaline, psilocybin
Solvents	Aerosol sprays, glue, toluene, gasoline, paint thinner
Over-the-counter drugs	Contain: atropine, scopolamine, antihistamines
Others	Phencyclidine (PCP), bromides

classifications, some of which are best used for research and some of which are the most pharmacologically correct. However, I present a breakdown of drugs into classes that have particular usefulness in clinical settings and where the drug class is determined by the most prominent CNS effects.[7]

This drug classification is presented in Table 1.1 along with some examples of the more frequently encountered drugs of each particular class. The divisions include:

1.4.1. General CNS Depressants

The most prominent effect of these drugs is depression of excitable tissues at all levels of the brain.[7] The CNS depressants include almost all sleeping medications, antianxiety drugs (also called minor tranquilizers), and alcohol. The antipsychotic drugs (also called major tranquilizers), such as chlorpromazine (Thorazine) or haloperidol (Haldol), are not CNS depressants, don't resemble the antianxiety drugs in their structures or predominant effects, are not physically addictive, and are rarely used to induce a "high."

1.4.2. CNS Sympathomimetics or Stimulants

The predominant effect of these drugs is stimulation of CNS tissues through blocking the actions of inhibitory nerve cells or by the release of transmitter substances (chemicals released from one brain cell to stimulate the next cell) from the cells, or by direct action of the drugs themselves. The substances most relevant to clinical situations include all the amphetamines, methylphenidate (Ritalin), and cocaine.

1.4.3. Opiate Analgesics

These drugs, also called *narcotic analgesics,* are used clinically to decrease pain, and they include morphine and other alkaloids of opium as well as synthetic morphinelike substances and semisynthetic opium derivatives. Prominent examples of these drugs include almost all pain-killing medications, ranging from propoxyphene (Darvon) to heroin.

1.4.4. The Cannabinols, or Marijuana

The active ingredient for all these substances is tetrahydrocannabinol, THC, with the predominant effect of producing euphoria, an altered time sense, and, at doses higher than those usually found in clinical situations, hallucinations. This is a "street" drug sold in the United States primarily as marijuana or hashish as pure THC is almost never sold on the streets (see Section 8.5.).

1.4.5. Psychedelics or Hallucinogens

The predominant effect of these substances is the production of hallucinations, usually of a visual nature. The hallucinogens have no accepted medical usefulness and are a second example of "street" drugs.

1.4.6. Solvents, Glues, and Aerosols

These substances are used in various fuels, aerosol sprays, glues, paints, and industrial solutions. They are used as drugs of abuse in attempts to alter the state of consciousness, producing primarily lightheadedness and confusion.

1.4.7. Over-the-Counter Drugs

A variety of substances are marketed for sale without prescription in the treatment of constipation, pain, nervousness, insomnia, etc. The sedative or hypnotic medications are the most frequently abused and contain atropine-type drugs (anticholinergics) and/or antihistamines and are taken to give feelings of lightheadedness and euphoria.

1.5. ALTERNATE CLASSIFICATION SCHEMES

An additional breakdown of these substances, addressing a series of "schedules" developed by the federal government, is presented in Table 1.2.[8,9] The classification is based on both the degree of medical usefulness and the abuse potential of the substance, ranging from Schedule I, which

Table 1.2
Drug Schedules with Examples[8,9]

Schedule I (High abuse, low usefulness):
   Examples: Heroin
          Hallucinogens
          Marijuana

Schedule II:
   Examples: Opium or morphine
          Codeine
          Sympathetic opiates (e.g., meperidine [Demerol])
          Barbiturates
          Amphetamines or methylphenidate (Ritalin)
          Methaqualone (Quaalude)

Schedule III:
   Examples: Aspirin with codeine
          Paregoric
          Methyprylon (Noludar)
          Glutethimide (Doriden)

Schedule IV:
   Examples: Phenobarbital
          Chloral hydrate (Noctec)
          Ethchlorvynol (Placidyl)
          Flurazepam (Dalmane)

Schedule V (Low abuse, high usefulness):
   Examples: Cheracol with codeine
          Robitussin A-C
          Terpin hydrate with codeine

includes those drugs with few accepted medical uses and a high abuse potential (e.g., heroin), to Schedule V, drugs that have a high level of medical usefulness and little known abuse potential. Unfortunately, it is not always possible to generalize from the schedule level to the actual drug effects, as exemplified by the classification of marijuana and heroin at the same level, and ethchlorvynol (Placidyl) and glutethimide (Doriden) in different categories despite their marked medicinal and abuse similarities.

Another way of looking at these drugs is to attempt to classify them by their "street" names. These differ between locales and within the same place over time; therefore, Table 1.3 can be seen as only a brief list of some of the more relevant street names that are *usually* used. It is important to gain some knowledge of the specific use of drug names in your vicinity. In the table, drugs are divided into the major classes outlined in this chapter, and the street names are given alphabetically within each class. For ease of reference, this is one of the rare places in this text where trade names rather than generic names are used.

Table 1.3
A Brief List of "Street" Drug Names

CNS Depressants[a]

Blue birds	Green and whites (Librium)	Seccy
Blue devil	Greenies	Seggy
Blue heaven	Nembies	Sleepers
Blues	Peanuts	T-bird
Bullets	Peter (chloral hydrate)	Toolies
Dolls[r]	Rainbows	Trangs (Librium type)
Double trouble	Red birds	Yellow jackets
Downs	Red devils	Yellows
Goofballs	Roaches (Librium)[r]	

Stimulants[b]

Bennies	Double cross	Roses
Blue angels	Flake (cocaine)	Snow (cocaine)
Chris	Footballs	Speed
Christine	Gold dust (cocaine)	Speedball
Christmas trees	Green and clears	(heroin plus cocaine)
Coast to coast	Hearts	Truck drivers
Coke (cocaine)	Lip poppers	Uppers
Co-pilot	Meth	Ups
Crisscross	Oranges	Wake ups
Crossroads	Peaches	Whites
Crystal (IV Methamphetamine)[r]	Pep pills	
Dexies	Pinks	

Analgesics

Heroin		Other	
Brown	Scat	Black (opium)	PG, or PO (Paregoric)
H	Shit	Blue velvet (Paregoric plus	Pinks and grays (Darvon)
H and stuff	Skag	antihistamine)	Poppy (opium)
Horse	Smack	Dollies (methadone)	Tar (opium)
Junk		M (morphine)	Terp (Terpin hydrate or
		Microdots (morphine)	cough syrup with codeine)

Cannabinols

Marijuanalike			Hashishlike (more potent)
Acapulco gold	MJ	Yesca	Bhang
Brick	Muggles		Charas
Grass	Pot		Gage
Hay	Reefer		Ganja
Hemp	Roach[r]		Hash
Jive	Rope		Rope
Joint	Sativa		Sweet Lucy
Key, or kee	Stick		
Lid	Tea		
Locoweed	Texas tea		
Mary Jane	Weed		

Hallucinogens		
Acid (LSD)	Cube (LSD)	Mescal (mescaline)
Angel dust (PCP)	D (LSD)	Owsleys (LSD)
Blue dots (LSD)	Hog (PCP)	Peace pill (PCP)
Cactus (mescaline)	LBJ (PCP)	Pearly gates (morning
Crystal[c]		glory seeds)

[a]Moderate length of action *like* secobarbital unless otherwise noted.
[b]A form of amphetamine unless otherwise stated.
[c]Multiple drugs have the same name.

1.6. A CLASSIFICATION OF DRUG PROBLEMS

All drugs of abuse cause intoxication, each induces psychological dependence (whatever that might be), and all are self-administered by an individual to change a level of consciousness or to increase his psychological comfort. Each class of drugs has its dangers, with patterns of problems differing between drug classes. In this introductory section, I'll present some general concepts that will be discussed in greater depth in each chapter.

There is a limited range of adverse reactions for the drugs of abuse, and it is thus possible to create a summary table of drug categories and the problems most prominent for each (see Table 1.4). This section of the chapter expands upon the information in the table. For most types of problems (e.g., a panic), I will first discuss the most usual history, then note the usual physical signs and symptoms and the most prominent psychological difficulties, and finally give an overview of relevant laboratory tests. The generalizations presented for panic reactions, flash-

Table 1.4
Most Clinically Significant Drug Problems by Class

	Panic	Flashbacks	Toxic	Psychosis	OBS	Withdrawal
Depressants	−	−	++	++	++	++
Stimulants	+	−	+	++	+	+
Opiates	−	−	++	−	+	++
Cannabinols	+	+	+	−	+	−
Hallucinogens	++	++	+	+	+	−
Solvents	−	−	+	−	++	−
Phencyclidine	+	?	++	++	++	?

backs, psychosis, and organic brain syndromes are so constant among drug categories that only a brief discussion of the clinical picture is presented within each relevant chapter. On the other hand, the toxic reactions and withdrawal pictures seen with the different drug classes are so distinct that detailed discussions of the clinical picture are presented within each chapter.

It is important at this juncture to note that, with the exception of toxicologic screens of the urine (telling *if* the drug has been taken in the last day to week) and blood (telling *how much* of the substance, if any, is in the blood), there are few laboratory tests that help to establish a drug diagnosis. The normal laboratory result for each of the toxicologic screens is at or near zero, and the normal values for most other blood tests (e.g., lactic dehydrogenase [LDH]) differ so much between laboratories that the reader should check with his own facility to determine what normal range is expected. A brief guide to the most usual normal test results is given in Table 1.5, and some positive blood toxicology results appear in Table 1.6.

Table 1.5
A Brief List of Relevant Lab Tests and Usual Norms

Abbreviation	Name	Usual value
	Chemistry	
	Amylase	35–160 (Somogyi) units
	Bilirubin	Total ≤ 1.0 mg/dl
		Direct ≤ 0.2 mg/dl
BSP	Bromsulphalein	< 5% retention at 45 minutes
BUN	Blood urea nitrogen	8.0–23.0 mg/dl
Ca	Calcium	9.0–10.6 mg/dl
	Creatinine	0.8–1.2 mg/dl
CPK	Creatinine phosphokinase	0–140 U/l
	Glucose	70–110 mg/dl
LDH	Lactic dehydrogenase	36–200 U/l
Mg	Magnesium	1.8–2.5 mg/dl
K	Potassium	3.5–4.5 mEq/l
SGOT	Serum glutamic oxalacetic transaminase	8–30 U/l
SGPT	Serum glutamic pyruvic transaminase	5–35 U/l
Na	Sodium	135–145 mEq/l
	Blood counts	
Hgb	Hemoglobin	Men: 14–18 gm
		Women: 12–16 gm
Hct	Hematocrit	Men: 42–52%
		Women: 37–47%
MCV	Mean corpuscular volume	Volume 82–92 μm^3
WBC	White blood cell count	$4.3 - 10.8 \times 10^3$ cells

Table 1.6
A Brief List of Relevant Blood Toxicologies

Drug	Toxic blood level	Units
Bromide	10–20	mEq/l
Chlordiazepoxide (Librium)	0.6–2.0	mg/dl
Diazepam (Valium)	0.5	mg/dl
Ethchlorvynol (Placidyl)	1.5–10.0	mg/dl
Glutethimide (Doriden)	1.0–3.0	mg/dl
Meperidine (Demerol)	100–500	μg/dl
Meprobamate (Miltown, Equanil)	5.0–10.0	mg/dl
Morphine	0.1–0.5	mg/dl
Oxazepam (Serax)	0.5–1.5	mg/dl
Phenobarbital	3–10	mg/dl

1.6.1. Panic Reaction

1.6.1.1. The Typical History

The patient is usually a first-time user who has typically taken marijuana, a hallucinogen, or stimulant.[10] Shortly after ingestion of the drug and the onset of the "typical" drug effects, the individual acutely develops fears that he is losing control, that he has done physical harm to himself, or that he is going crazy, and he is brought in for help by friends, relatives, or the police.

1.6.1.2. Physical Signs and Symptoms

Physical findings reflect fear, anxiety, and sympathetic nervous system overactivity (for example, increased pulse and respiratory rates) occurring in the midst of a panic. This overactivity includes an elevated pulse (usually about 120 beats per minute), an elevated respiratory rate (over 20 or 25 per minute), and an elevated blood pressure. The patient may also demonstrate slightly dilated pupils and excess perspiration.

1.6.1.3. Psychological State

Fear of going crazy, developing uncontrollable behavior, or the occurrence of permanent brain or heart damage (e.g., having a heart attack) dominate the clinical picture.

1.6.1.4. Relevant Laboratory Tests

Depending on the patient's clinical picture, steps must be taken to rule out any obvious physical pathology. Thus, in addition to establishing the level of vital signs, it is necessary to evaluate the need for an *electrocardiogram* (EKG) and to draw routine baseline laboratory studies (e.g., red blood cell count [RBC], glucose, liver and kidney function tests, white blood cell count [WBC], tests of skeletal or heart muscle damage such as creatinine phosphokinase [CPK], etc.). Some of the more relevant tests along with their abbreviations and *most usual* normal values are presented in Table 1.5. Of course, when a drug reaction is suspected but no adequate history can be obtained, urine (approximately 50 ml) and/or blood (approximately 20 ml) should be sent to the laboratory for a toxicologic screen to determine which, if any, drugs are present.

1.6.2. Flashback

A flashback, also most frequently seen with the cannabinols and the hallucinogens, is the unwanted recurrence of drug effects. This is probably a heterogeneous group of problems, including the presence of residual drug in the body, psychological stress, a behavioral "panic," or the possibility of a temporary alteration in brain functioning.

1.6.2.1. The Typical History

This picture is most frequently seen after the repeated use of marijuana or hallucinogens. The typical patient gives a history of past drug use with no recent intake to explain the episode of feeling "high."

1.6.2.2. Physical Signs and Symptoms

These depend on how the patient responds to the flashback, that is, his degree of "panic." Physical pathology is usually minimal and ranges from no physical symptoms to a full-blown panic as described above.

1.6.2.3. Psychological State

The patient most typically complains of a mild altered time sense or visual hallucinations (e.g., bright lights, geometric objects, or a "trailing" seen when objects move). Symptoms are most common when the subject enters darkness or before he goes to sleep. The emotional reaction may be one of perplexity or a paniclike fear of brain damage or of going crazy.

1.6.2.4. Relevant Laboratory Tests

Except for the unusually intense or atypical case where actual brain damage might be considered (this would require a brain wave tracing or electroencephalogram [EEG], an adequate neurologic examination, X rays of the skull, etc.), there are no specific laboratory tests. The patient will probably be drug-free, and it is likely that even toxicologic screens will not be helpful.

1.6.3. Toxic Reaction

A toxic reaction is really an overdose occurring when an individual has taken so much of the drug that the body support systems no longer work properly. Clinically, this is most frequently seen with the CNS depressants and opiates. A detailed discussion of this phenomenon is given within each relevant chapter, as the picture differs markedly among drug types.

1.6.4. Psychosis

Psychosis, as used here, occurs when an awake and alert individual loses contact with reality.

1.6.4.1. The Typical History

Drug-induced psychoses are usually seen in individuals who have repeatedly consumed CNS depressants, over-the-counter or prescription atropinelike drugs, stimulants, hallucinogens, or phencyclidine (PCP). The onset of symptoms is usually abrupt (within minutes to hours) and represents a gross change from the person's normal level of functioning. The disturbance is dramatic and may result in the patient's being brought to the emergency room by the police.

1.6.4.2. Physical Signs and Symptoms

There are few physical symptoms that are typical of any particular psychotic state. It is the loss of contact with reality occurring during intoxication that dominates the picture. However, during the psychosis, an individual may be quite upset and present with a rapid pulse or an elevated blood pressure.

1.6.4.3. Psychological State

A psychosis occurs with the development of either hallucinations (an unreal sensory input, such as seeing things) or a delusion (an unreal and fixed thought into which the individual has no insight). In general, the drug-induced psychotic state lasts for a day to at most a week and is usually totally reversible. As will be discussed in greater depth in the specific chapters, there is little evidence, if any, of chronic or permanent psychoses being induced in individuals who have shown no obvious psychopathology antedating their drug experience.

1.6.4.4. Relevant Laboratory Tests

No specific laboratory findings are associated with the psychosis, as the patient may be drug-free and still out of contact with reality. For patients who abuse drugs intravenously, the stigmata of infection (e.g., a high WBC) and hepatitis (e.g., elevated SGOT, SGPT, CPK, and LDH) may be seen. It is also *possible* that a urine or blood toxicologic screen will reveal evidence of a drug.

1.6.5. Organic Brain Syndrome

An organic brain syndrome (OBS) consists of confusion, disorientation, and decreased intellectual functioning.

1.6.5.1. The Typical History

Any drug can induce a state of confusion and/or disorientation (an OBS) if given in high enough doses, but at very high levels, the physical signs and symptoms of a toxic overdose predominate. There are a number of drugs, including the atropinelike substances, the CNS depressants and PCP, that produce confusion at relatively low doses. There are, in addition, some factors that predispose a person to confusion, including physical debilitation (e.g., hepatitis), advanced age, a history of prior head trauma, or a long history of drug or alcohol abuse. These factors combine to explain the varied types of onset for organicities ranging from a very rapidly developing picture after PCP in a healthy young man to a slow onset (e.g., over days to weeks) of increasing organicity for an elderly individual taking even therapeutic levels of CNS depressants.

1.6.5.2. Physical Signs and Symptoms

As defined in this text, the OBS patient most often presents with a stable physical condition and a predominance of mental pathology. However, because an organicity is more likely to be seen in an individual with some sort of physical problem, any mixture of physical signs and symptoms can be seen.

1.6.5.3. Psychological State

The patient demonstrates confusion about where he is, what he is doing there, the proper date and time, or who he is. He has trouble understanding concepts and assimilating new ideas but usually maintains some insight into the fact that his mind is not working properly. This, in turn, may result in a level of fear or irritability. The signs of an OBS may be accompanied by visual or tactile (i.e., feeling) hallucinations.

1.6.5.4. Relevant Laboratory Tests

While the OBS may continue beyond the length of action of any drug (especially in the elderly), a blood or urine toxicologic screen may be helpful. It's also important to rule out aggressively all potentially reversible nondrug causes of confusion. Thus, in addition to a good neurologic examination, blood tests should be drawn to determine the status of the electrolytes (especially sodium, calcium, and potassium [see Table 1.5]), blood counts, (especially the hematocrit and hemoglobin levels, as shown in the table), liver and kidney function tests (including the BUN and creatinine for the kidney and the SGOT, SGPT, and LDH for the liver). It is also necessary to evaluate the need for skull X rays (to look for fractures and signs of internal bleeding), a spinal tap (to rule out bleeding, infection, or tumors of the CNS), and an EEG (to look for focal problems as well as general brain functioning).

1.6.6. Withdrawal or Abstinence Syndrome

The withdrawal or abstinence syndrome consists of the development of physiological and psychological symptoms when a physically addicting drug is stopped too quickly. The length of the withdrawal syndrome varies directly with the half-life (the time necessary to metabolize one-half after drug dose) of the drug, and the intensity of the reaction depends upon the drug itself, the usual dose taken, and the length of time over which the drug was administered. Clinically significant withdrawal syndromes are seen for the CNS depressants, the opiates, and the stimulants. Because these syndromes differ for each specific kind of drug, I have *not* presented general rules here but rather refer the reader to the relevant chapter.

1.7. A GENERAL INTRODUCTION TO EMERGENCY AND CRISIS TREATMENT

The emergency care of the drug-abusing patient is covered within each chapter and in a general review in Chapter 12. The treatment approaches represent common-sense applications of those lessons learned about the drug category, the probable natural course of that class of difficulty, and the dictum of "First do no harm."

1.7.1. Acute Emergency Care[11]

One must first address the life-threatening problems that may be associated with toxic reactions, psychoses, organic brain syndromes, withdrawal, and medical problems. The approach to emergency care begins by first establishing an adequate airway, supporting circulation and controlling hemorrhage, and dealing with any life-threatening behavior.

1.7.2. Evaluation

After the patient has been stabilized, it is important to carry out evaluations of other serious problems through gathering a good history from the patient and/or a resource person (usually a relative), doing careful physical and neurologic examinations, and performing the relevant laboratory tests.

1.7.3. Subacute Care

1. It is then possible to begin the more subacute care, attempting to keep medications to a minimum, especially for symptoms of *panic* and *flashbacks*, which tend to respond to reassurance.

2. For *toxic reactions*, the subacute goal is supporting vital signs until the body has had a chance to metabolize the ingested substance adequately.

3. The transient nature of the *psychoses* indicates that the best care is suppression of any destructive behavior during the several days necessary for the patient to recover.

4. Evaluation of an *OBS* requires carefully diagnosing and treating all life-threatening causes.

5. *Withdrawal* is usually treated through an adequate physical evaluation to rule out associated medical disorders, giving rest and good nutrition, and slowly decreasing the level of the addictive substances.

6. *Medical problems* must be handled individually.

1.8. ONWARD

You have now been introduced to my general philosophy involving drugs, drug problems, and their treatment. I now proceed with a detailed discussion of the CNS depressants, which is followed by two chapters on alcohol and the treatment of alcoholism, serving as a prototype for the remaining chapters in the text. Each of the clinically relevant drug types is then discussed, with the two final chapters emphasizing emergency problems of substance misusers in general and an introduction to rehabilitation.

REFERENCES

1. Fingl, E., & Woodbury, D. M. Chapter 1: General principles. In L. S. Goodman & A. Gilman (Eds.), *The Pharmacological Basis of Therapeutics*. New York: Macmillan, 1975, pp. 1–46.
2. Cohen, S. (Ed.). Pharmacology of drugs of abuse. *Drug Abuse and Alcoholism Newsletter*. 5(6):1–4, 1976.

3. Alford, G. S., & Alford, H. F. Benzodiazepine-induced state-dependent learning: A correlative of abuse potential? *Addictive Behaviors.* 1:261–267, 1976.
4. Jaffe, J. H. Chapter 16: Drug addiction and drug abuse. In L. S. Goodman & A. Gilman (Eds.), *The Pharmacological Basis of Therapeutics.* New York: Macmillan, 1975, pp. 284–324.
5. Siegel, S. Evidence from rats that morphine tolerance is a learned response. *Journal of Comparative and Physiological Psychology.* 89(5):498–506, 1975.
6. Parker, L. F., & Radow, B. Morphine-like physical dependence: A pharmacologic method for drug assessment using the rat. *Pharmacology Biochemistry and Behavior.* 2:613–618, 1974.
7. Franz, D. N. Section II: Drugs acting on the central nervous system. Introduction. In L. S. Goodman & A. Gilman (Eds.), *The Pharmacological Basis of Therapeutics.* New York: Macmillan, 1975, pp. 47–52.
8. Konner, D. D. *Controlled Substances Inventory List.* Washington, D.C.: U.S. Dept. of Justice, Jan. 1977.
9. Cohen, S. (Ed.). The drug schedules: An updating for professionals. *Drug Abuse and Alcoholism Newsletter.* 5(3):1–4, 1976.
10. Weil, A. T. Adverse reactions to marihuana. Classification and suggested treatment. *New England Journal of Medicine* 5(3):1–4, 1976.
11. Boedeker, E.C., & Dauber, J. H. (Eds.). *Manual of Medical Therapeutics,* 21st Ed. Boston: Little, Brown, 1974.

CHAPTER 2

The CNS Depressants

2.1. INTRODUCTION

The central nervous system (CNS) depressant drugs include a variety of medications, such as hypnotics, antianxiety drugs (also called minor tranquilizers), and alcohol. The general anesthetics will not be discussed here, as time and space constraints force me to limit the discussion to the substances most clinically important in drug abuse. One anesthetic agent, phencyclidine (PCP), is abused as a hallucinogen and is discussed in Section 8.3.

The CNS depressants all have clinical usefulness and most have an abuse potential. When used alone, they cause an intoxication or "high" similar to alcohol, but they can also be mixed with other drugs, such as stimulants, in attempts to modify some of the effects or side effects of those drugs.

As indicated by the high rate of prescriptions, a major avenue of supply is through the physician. In addition, many of the legally manufactured depressants find their way into the street marketplace.

The prototypical depressant drug is the barbiturate. These medications have been available since the 1806s[1] and have been prescribed for a wide variety of problems. The generic names of all barbiturates in the United States end in *-al*, and in Britain in *-one*.[1]

2.1.1. Pharmacology

2.1.1.1. General Characteristics

The different CNS depressants possess markedly different lengths of action, as discussed below. Blood levels depend upon physical redistribution of the drug between various parts of the body, metabolic breakdown of the substance (usually in the liver), and excretion via the kidneys.

2.1.1.2. Predominant Effects

The specific pharmacologic mechanisms by which these drugs exert their effects are not completely known, but theories are discussed in other texts.[1] The depressants result in reversible depression of the activity of all excitable tissues—especially those of the CNS—with greatest effects on the synapse (the space between two nerve cells).[1,2] The resulting depression in activity ranges from a slight lethargy or sleepiness, through various levels of anesthesia, to death from breathing and heart depression. It should be noted that, paradoxically, the hypnotics and the anti-anxiety drugs sometimes cause extreme excitement when given to children and elderly patients (a *paradoxical reaction*).

2.1.1.3. Tolerance and Dependence

2.1.1.3.1. Tolerance

The tolerance to these drugs is clincially important and occurs through both increased metabolism of the drug after its administration (*drug dispositional* or *metabolic tolerance*) and through apparent adaptation of the CNS to the presence of the drug (*pharmacodynamic tolerance*).[1] However, metabolic tolerance also results in the enhanced metabolism of a variety of other substances, including the anticoagulant medications, with resulting altered blood levels. As is true with all medications, tolerance is not an all-or-none phenomenon, and most individuals do not demonstrate enhanced toleration to lethal doses of the depressants (with the possible exception of alcohol).[2]

An important aspect of tolerance occurs with concomitant administration of additional depressant drugs. If the second drug is administered alone, cross-tolerance will probably be seen, at least in part, because of the expansion of the liver's capacity to metabolize depressant drugs. However, if the second depressant drug is administered at the same time as the first, the two drugs compete for metabolism within the liver, neither is metabolized properly, and the toxic effects of one drug appear to multiply the toxic effects of the second. Therefore, even an individual with tolerance to one drug can have a fatal overdose with a concomitantly administered second drug, a common clinical circumstance with barbiturates and alcohol.

2.1.1.3.2. Dependence

All CNS depressants, including the benzodiazepines like chlordiazepoxide (Librium) and diazepam (Valium) (although they probably have the least potential to produce the syndrome of any of the drugs) produce a withdrawal state when stopped abruptly after the relatively continuous administration of high doses. The withdrawal picture *resembles* a rebound hyperexcitability characterized by body changes in a direction opposite to those seen with the administration of the drug (this may not be the actual pharmacologic mechanism).[2] In general, concomitant misuse of more than one depressant drug (again, an example is alcohol plus a barbiturate) increases the predisposition toward withdrawal.

It is possible to see signs of withdrawal after several weeks of intoxication,[2] but, in general, the severity of the withdrawal syndrome parallels the strength of the drug, the doses taken, and the length of administration.[3] The actual dosage varies with the drug and the individual, but for a drug like pentobarbital, for example, administration of 400 mg a day for three months results in definite withdrawal EEG changes in at least one-third of the individuals taking the drug; 600 mg for one to two months results in a mild to moderate level of withdrawal in half of the individuals, with 10% going on to severe withdrawal, including seizures; and 900 mg for two months results in seizures in 75% of the individuals, with most demonstrating a confusion-disorientation syndrome (organic brain syndrome [OBS]).[2] With a drug like meprobamate (Miltown or Equanil), one can see severe withdrawal in an individual taking three to six grams daily over 40 days. As a general rule, abuse of 500 mg of a barbiturate or an equivalent dose of other drugs will result in a risk for withdrawal seizures.[4] For the benzodiazepines, minor to moderate withdrawal symptoms can be seen with individuals taking two or three times the usual clinical dose for only 16 weeks.[5,6]

2.1.1.4. Specific Drugs

Table 2.1 gives numerous examples of members of the different classes of hypnotic and antianxiety drugs. The actions of members of two major subclasses of drugs overlap greatly. For example, antianxiety drugs in high enough doses induce sleep, while the hypnotics, for many years, were labeled *hypnosedatives* and administered to treat anxiety. In addition, some of the hypnotics are used as general anesthetic agents, and the antianxiety drugs have muscle-relaxing properties that are used to treat muscle spasms and to help carry out diagnostic procedures such as bronchoscopy or endoscopy (passing a tube through the mouth to allow direct observation of the lining of the bronchial tree or the stomach).

2.1.1.4.1. The Hypnotics

As shown in Table 2.1, the most commonly used substances are the barbiturates, the barbituratelike drugs, and two other hypnotics.

Table 2.1
CNS Depressants

Drug type	Generic name	Trade name
HYPNOTICS		
Barbiturates		
Ultra-short-acting	Thiopental	Pentothal
	Methohexital	Brevital
Intermediate-acting	Pentobarbital	Nembutal
	Secobarbital	Seconal
	Amobarbital	Amytal
	Butabarbital	Butisol
Long-acting	Phenobarbital	Luminal
Barbituratelike		
	Methaqualone	Quāalude
	Ethchlorvynol	Placidyl
	Methyprylon	Noludar
	Glutethimide	Doriden
Others		
	Flurazepam	Dalmane
	Chloral hydrate	Noctec
ANTIANXIETY DRUGS		
Benzodiazepines		
	Chlordiazepoxide	Librium
	Diazepam	Valium
	Oxazepam	Serax
	Chlorazepate	Tranxene
Carbamates		
	Meprobamate	Miltown
		Equanil
	Tybamate	Salacen
		Tybatran

1. The first subclass of *barbiturates* consists of the rarely abused *ultrashort* drugs (used to induce anesthesia) with lengths of action of minutes (e.g., sodium pentothal and hexobarbital). The *short-to-intermediate*–acting barbiturates exert their major effect for a period of approximately four hours, making them ideal for helping people to get to sleep. These include the drugs most frequently prescribed and abused as hypnotics, such as secobarbital (Seconal) and pentobarbital (Nembutal). Finally, the *long-lasting* drugs, exemplified by phenobarbital, are most often used to treat chronic conditions such as epilepsy. These drugs are relatively rarely abused.

2. The *barbituratelike drugs* (e.g., glutethimide [Doriden] and methaqualone [Quāalude]) were almost all introduced as "nonaddictive

and safe" substitutes for the barbiturates. They were developed in an attempt to overcome some of the drawbacks of barbiturate hypnotics, such as the morning-after "hangover," residual sleepiness, drug-induced disturbances in sleep patterns (especially rapid eye movement [REM] sleep), and the highly lethal overdose potential of barbiturates. However, most barbiturate-like hypnotics share the dangers of the barbiturates. Two drugs are *especially* dangerous in overdoses as they are highly fat-soluble and resistant to excretion, offer few clinical advantages, and should be prescribed rarely, if at all. These are ethchlorvynol (Placidyl) and glutethimide (Doriden).[7] Another drug, methaqualone (Quāalude) has been especially widely abused.[8]

3. The third and final group of hypnotics discussed here is exemplifed by paraldehyde and chloral hydrate (Noctec), drugs that share most of the dangers outlined for the barbiturate and barbituratelike hypnotics. The third drug, representing the only departure from these general drawbacks, is the benzodiazepine flurazepam (Dalmane). While this drug does disturb sleep patterns,[9] the ratio between its effective dose and the lethal overdose is huge, making it relatively safe.

4. In summary, the hypnotics share serious drawbacks. They disturb the natural sleep pattern, they are extremely dangerous if taken as an overdose (with the probable exception of flurazepam), and all have an abuse potential. Several of the drugs, ethchlorvynol and glutethimide, have additional dangers of delayed metabolism, which make their prescription even more dangerous than that of the usual drug.

It appears that all hypnotic medications lose their effectiveness if taken nightly for more than two weeks.[10] Therefore, considering their potential as suicide agents and their limited time of efficacy when used daily, there is a serious question about the wisdom of prescribing these medications for anything more than a short-term, acute crisis. If a hypnotic is required for an acute anxiety situation, I use flurazepam (Dalmane), but never for more than two weeks at a time.

Numerous other approaches to handling insomnia are available and are discussed in detail in other texts.[11] For instance, after carefully ruling out problems to which insomnia might be secondary,[12] I prescribe a schedule of going to bed and getting up at the same time each day, no caffeinated beverages, and no naps. Milk at bedtime can be a useful adjunct, perhaps because of its tryptophan content.

2.1.1.4.2. The Antianxiety Drugs

The two classes of drugs most frequently prescribed for anxiety are the benzodiazepines (e.g., diazepam, or Valium) and the carbamates (e.g., meprobamate, or Equanil) as shown in Table 2.1. These drugs have been demonstrated to be highly effective in handling *acute* anxiety,[13] but no well-controlled study has yet proven that their efficacy lasts more than a month when taken daily.

The major dangers include a disturbance in sleep pattern and a change in affect (increased irritability, hostility, and lethargy). In addition, while the benzodiazepines have a very wide range between therapeutic and lethal doses, the carbamates are lethal when taken in overdosage. Most members of these two drug subclasses have a length of action that exceeds the usual time between administration of doses, with the possible result of accumulation of these drugs in the body (the one exception is oxazepam [Serax]). I never prescribe the carbamates (Miltown, Equanil, or Tybamate), because of their much higher addictive potential and greater possibility of fatal overdosage when compared to benzodiazepines.

2.1.2. Epidemiology and Pattern of Abuse

The CNS depressants are prescribed in great quantities, as approximately 90% of hospitalized medical/surgical patients receive orders for hypnotic and/or antianxiety medication during their inpatient stay,[14] and in excess of 15% of American adults use these drugs during any one year.[15] Thus, it is not surprising that it has been estimated that up to 10% of general medical/surgical patients and 30% of individuals with serious psychiatric histories have, at some time, *felt* psychologically dependent on antianxiety or hypnotic drugs,[16] with outright abuse seen for between 5% and 10%.[17,18]

In simple terms, depressant drug abusers fall into the two classes of those who receive the drugs on prescription and those who (belonging to a "street culture") primarily misuse illegally obtained medications. One survey has revealed that between one-fourth and one-third of abusers of illegally obtained medications report using hypnotics or antianxiety drugs over the prior month,[19] usually periodic ingestion of 30–80 mg of diazepam (Valium), frequently in combination with other drugs. For both types of abusers, at least 10% of all "drug mentions" in emergency rooms and crisis clinics are of diazepam.[20]

Thus, misuse of these drugs should be considered in the evaluation of almost any patient seen in a usual medical setting, an emergency room, or a crisis clinic. In light of the limited time that these medications stay effective when taken daily, there is rarely a valid clinical need to prescribe them for more than two weeks.

2.1.3. Establishing the Diagnosis

Identification of the individual misusing or abusing CNS depressants requires a high index of suspicion, especially for patients with an OBS or paranoid delusions and for all patients who insist upon receiving prescriptions for any of these medications. It is imperative that these drugs not be given to patients who are not known to the physician, and that, when they are prescribed, only relatively small samples be given (both to decrease the suicide overdose potential[21] and to discourage misuse), that no "repeats" be allowed, that bottles be labeled as to contents, and that past records be evaluated to determine how long the patient has been on the medication.

2.2. EMERGENCY PROBLEMS

The outline given below follows the general format presented in Table 1.3, reviewing the possible areas of difficulty seen in emergency rooms, the outpatient office, and crisis clinics. The most common problems seen for the depressants are the toxic overdose, withdrawal, and the temporary psychosis.

2.2.1. Panic Reaction (See Sections 1.6.1., 5.2.1., 7.2.1., and 8.2.1.)

Panic reactions (high levels of anxiety due to the fear of either going crazy or coming to physical harm as a result of the normal effects of the drug) are most frequently seen with stimulants and hallucinogenic drugs. They are rarely noted as part of the reaction to sedating drugs, such as CNS depressants and opiates.

2.2.1.1. Clinical Picture

The closest one comes to seeing a panic reaction is the hyperexcitability (paradoxical reaction) seen in some children and elderly individuals receiving depressant drugs, where the patient is frightened and excited, can't sleep, and has excessive energy.[22] Problems begin in the first hour or so after taking the drug and remain for the length of action of the substance.

2.2.1.2. Treatment

In this instance, the clinical picture tends to clear within hours, with only general support and reassurance. It is best to avoid administering other drugs.

2.2.2. Flashbacks

These are not known to occur with CNS depressants. If a patient reports them, other diagnoses (especially emotional or neurologic diseases) should be considered.

2.2.3. Toxic Reactions (See Sections 4.2.3., 6.2.3., and 12.4.)

The most usual toxic reaction seen with the depressant drugs occurs with either a deliberate or an inadvertent overdose.

2.2.3.1. Clinical Picture

2.2.3.1.1. The History

The toxic reaction usually develops over a matter of hours, and the patient often presents in an obtunded state with or without evidence of recent drug ingestion. This reaction can be seen when an individual mixes depressants together (usually alcohol and hypnotics), develops a confused organic state that results in inadvertent repeated administration of the drug (an automatism[23]), unintentionally takes too high a dose of street drugs, or makes a deliberate attempt at suicide.

2.2.3.1.2. Physical Signs and Symptoms

Toxic reactions are characterized by various levels of anesthesia and decreased CNS, cardiac, and respiratory functioning. An overdose of a depressant drug is very serious. Physical signs must be carefully evaluated in a manner similar to that reported in Section 6.2.3., for opiates and as suggested by other authors.[24] Examination includes:

1. Careful evaluation of vital signs and reflexes, with the findings depending upon the drug dose, the time elapsed since ingestion, and any complicating brain conditions such as hypoxia.[24]

2. The neurologic exams will help establish the degree of coma. Important aspects include:

   a. *Pupillary reflexes*. Usually midpoint and slowly reactive, except with glutethimide (Doriden), where pupils tend to be enlarged.

   b. *Corneal reflexes*. Present only in mild coma.

   c. *Tendon reflexes and pain reflexes*. Tend to be depressed.[24]

3. Cardiac arrhythmias may be present, especially with the short-acting barbiturates.[24]

4. The lungs may be congested from heart failure or positional or infective pneumonia.

2.2.3.1.3. Psychological State

Because the patient often presents in a stupor or coma, there are usually few other distinctive psychological attributes.

2.2.3.1.4. Relevant Laboratory Tests (See Section 6.2.3.1.4.)

As with any shocklike state or comparable medical emergency, it is important to carefully monitor vital signs and blood gases (arterial oxygen and CO_2) to evaluate the need for a respirator. A toxicologic screen on either urine (50ml) or blood (10ml) should also be carried out to determine the specific drug involved and the amount of the substance in the blood, and baseline blood chemistries and blood counts should be taken as outlined in Table 1.5. If the cause of the stupor or coma is not obvious, a thorough neurological evaluation for ancillary damage (including an EEG, skull X rays, a spinal tap, etc.) must be done.

2.2.3.2. Treatment (See Section 6.2.3.2.)

Treatment begins with emergency procedures to guarantee an adequate airway, making sure that the heart is functioning, and dealing with any concomitant bleeding. The general goal is to support the vital signs until enough of the drug has been metabolized so that the patient is stable,[25] following the general approach presented in Table 2.2. The specific emergency maneuvers will depend upon the clinical status of the patient. These may range from simple observation for mild overdoses to starting an intravenous infusion (IV), placing the patient on a respirator, and admitting him to an intensive care unit. The steps, not given in a fixed order, include the following:[24]

1. Establish a *clear airway, intubate* (use an inflatable cuff in case you want to do a gastric lavage) if needed, and place on a *respirator* if necessary. The respirator should use compressed air (oxygen can decrease the respiratory drive) at a rate of 10–12 breaths per minute.

2. Evaluate the *cardiovascular status* and control *bleeding;* treat shock with plasma expanders, saline, Dextran, or the relevant drugs;[25] administer *external cardiac massage/defibrillation/intracardiac adrenaline,* if needed.

3. Begin an IV (large-gauge needle), replacing all fluid loss (e.g., urine), *plus* 20 ml for insensible loss (from respirations and perspiration), each hour.

4. Establish a means of measuring *urinary output* (bladder catheter, if needed). Send 50 ml of urine for a toxicologic screen.[25]

5. Carry out *gastric lavage* if oral medication was taken in the last 4–6 hours.[25] Carry out lavage with saline until you get a clear return. You may give 60 ml of *castor oil* via the stomach tube, especially if fat-soluble drugs like glutethimide (Doriden) were taken.[25]

6. Recognizing that analgesics can cause a similar picture and that the patient may have ingested more than one type of medication, consider the possiblity of a narcotic overdose. This is easily tested through

Table 2.2
Treatment of the Depressant Toxic Reaction

Diagnose	History, clinical signs
First steps	Airway, assist respiration
	Cardiac
	Check electrolytes
	Treat shock
	Lavage (use cuff if obtunded; activated charcoal; castor oil?)
Consider	Forced diuresis (limited value)
	Hemodialysis
Avoid	CNS stimulants

the administration of a narcotic antagonist such as *naloxone* (Narcan) at a dose of 0.4 ml, given either intramuscularly (IM) or IV. If the patient has ingested narcotic analgesics to the point of obtundation, a rapid reversal of the picture should be demonstrated.

7. Carry out a more thorough *physical* and *neurologic exam*. This must include *pupils, corneal reflexes, tendon reflexes,* presence of *pathologic reflexes* (e.g., snout reflex), *pain perception* (use Achilles tendon), and level of *awake/alert status*. (See Sections 6.2.3., and 12.4.)

8. Draw *bloods* for arterial blood gases, general blood tests to evaluate liver and kidney functioning, blood counts, and toxicologic screen.

9. Gather a thorough *history* of the following:

    a. Recent drugs (type, amount, time)
    b. Alcohol
    c. Chronic diseases
    d. Allergies
    e. Current treatments

Obtain this information from the patient and/or any available resource person.

10. For the comatose patient, protect against *decubital ulcers* by frequent turning, and *protect the eyes* by taping the lids closed if necessary.

11. Establish a *flow sheet* for the following:

    a. Vital signs
    b. Level of reflexes (number 7 above)
    c. Urinary output
    d. IV fluids

These should be recorded every 30 minutes. An example is given in a reference text.[4]

12. Consider *forced diuresis*. This is not needed for patients with stable vital signs and those who present deep tendon reflexes (e.g., Grade I or II coma[24]) and rarely helps for chlordiazepoxide hydrochloride (Librium) or diazepam (Valium).[4] If either diuresis or dialysis is used, special care must be taken to maintain proper electrolyte levels and to avoid precipitating congestive failure.

If diuresis is needed, you may use the following:

  a. Furosemide (Lasix), 40–120 mg, as often as needed to maintain 250 ml or more per hour.
  b. IV fluids can be used with the general approach being to give enough saline and water with glucose to maintain urinary output in excess of 250 ml per hour.

13. Hemodialysis or peritoneal dialysis can be considered for the patient in a deep coma, but this is rarely needed. Reasons for giving dialysis are discussed in Section 12.4.3.

14. Evaluate the need for *antibiotics*. Do *not* use these prophylactically.

15. Do *not* use CNS stimulants.

16. For the unresponsive patient who requires admission to an intensive care unit, it is possible to establish a prognosis by observing the levels and the degree of change in systolic pressure, the central venous pressure, and the acid–base balance (pH), as described in the reference.[25] A special word of warning is required regarding the ability of the depressant drugs to produce a temporary flat electroencephalogram (EEG) which reverses within a matter of days.[2]

17. There are some special CNS depressant pictures but most of these generalizations would hold for any drug. However, one might expect a longer period of coma with the fat-soluble drugs like glutethimide (Doriden) and ethchlorvynol (Placidyl). These patients can enter an emergency room looking alert or be treated in a hospital and appear to come out of their coma only to relapse into a deep level of obtundation.

2.2.4. Psychosis (See Sections 1.6.4., 4.2.4., and 5.2.4.)

2.2.4.1. The Clinical Picture

The depressant drugs can produce a temporary psychosis characterized by an acute onset, a clear sensorium (the patient is alert and oriented), auditory hallucinations, and/or paranoid delusions (e.g., thinking that someone is plotting against or trying to harm him). This picture has been more clearly described as it relates to alcohol and thus is discussed in greater depth in Section 4.2.4. It is probable that the generalizations presented for alcohol hold for the other depressants as well.

2.2.4.2. Treatment

The psychosis will probably clear within two days to two weeks with supportive care. Medications should not be given unless the paranoia and/or hallucinations create a serious danger to the patient or those around him. Then, antipsychotic drugs—e.g., haloperidol (Haldol), 1–5 mg four times a day (QID)—can be used *until* the clinical picture clears.

2.2.5. Organic Brain Syndrome (See Section 1.6.5.)

The OBS can result as part of intoxication or an *overdose,* or during withdrawal. The confusion associated with intoxication tends to be mild and transient and thus will not be discussed here.

2.2.5.1. Overdose

2.2.5.1.1. Clinical Picture

An overdose short of a coma can produce confusion, disorientation, decreased mentation, and impaired memory-processing. This picture closely resembles that seen during high-level alcohol intoxication. It may develop at even low doses in individuals at high risk for confusion, such as the elderly.[28, 29]

2.2.5.1.2. Treatment

The confusional state is best treated with observation, usually in an inpatient setting where the patient is protected from wandering or harming himself. For younger individuals, the confusion usually clears within a matter of hours to days, but for older people it might require an extended period of treatment of two weeks or longer. In either instance, it is best to avoid concomitant administration of any drug.

2.2.5.2. Withdrawal

2.2.5.2.1. Clinical Picture

A rapidly evolving OBS can be seen during withdrawal from these drugs. It is usually temporary, rarely lasting more than a few days even without treatment. When it develops, one must take care to rule out other potentially lethal causes of OBS, including trauma, occult bleeding, or brain damage.

2.2.5.2.2. Treatment

This is discussed in Section 2.2.6.2.

2.2.6. Drug Withdrawal Syndrome (See Sections 4.2.6., and 6.2.6.)

The depressant withdrawal syndrome consists of a constellation of symptoms that *might* develop in an individual taking any of these drugs daily in excessive doses. The final clinical picture is usually a mixture of any or all of the possible symptoms, running a time course that tends to last three to seven days for the short-acting drugs (the most frequently abused CNS depressants[30]), but it may be longer for longer-acting drugs like diazepam (Valium).

2.2.6.1. The Clinical Picture

2.2.6.1.1. History

A CNS depressant withdrawal syndrome must be considered in any individual who presents with autonomic nervous system dysfunction along with agitation and who asks the physician for a CNS depressant drug. This syndrome can be seen in both the "street" addict, who may be abusing the drug either orally or IV, and the middle-class abuser who obtains the drug on prescription but takes more than prescribed. The syndrome begins slowly over a period of hours and may not peak until Day 2 or 3.

The time course for withdrawal for barbiturates, such as pentobarbital, or a drug like meprobamate (Miltown or Equanil) is outlined in Table 2.3. This table can be used as a general outline for what might be expected, showing the beginning of symptoms within a half day of stopping or decreasing the medications, a peak intensity at 24–72 hours, and a disappearance of acute symptoms sometime before Day 7. The time course of withdrawal is probably a good deal longer for the longer-acting barbiturates and the antianxiety drugs, such as chlordiazepoxide (Librium), where it has been reported that seizures and delirium can begin as late as Day 7 or 8.[3]

2.2.6.1.2. Physical Signs and Symptoms

The withdrawal symptomatology consists of a strong mixture of both psychological and physical problems. The patient usually develops a fine *tremor, gastrointestinal (GI) upset, muscle aches,* and problems of the *autonomic nervous system* (e.g., increased rates for pulse and respiration, a fever, and a labile blood pressure). With any CNS depressant, but especially the barbiturates, somewhere between 5% and perhaps 20% of the

Table 2.3
Time Course of Acute Withdrawal for
Short/Intermediate Barbiturates and Meprobamate[2-4, 30-32]

Time (after last dose)	Symptom	Severity
12–16 hours	Intoxicated state *Onset:* Anxiety, tremors, anorexia, weakness, nausea/vomiting, cramps, hypotension, increased reflexes	Mild
24 hours	Weakness, tremors, increased reflexes, increased pleading for drug	Mild
	High risk for grand mal seizures Delirium	Severe
24–72 hours	Peak intensity	
3–7 days	Symptoms gradually disappear	
1 week–6 months	Some anxiety, sleep disturbance, autonomic nervous system irregularities	Mild

individuals will develop grand mal *convulsions*—usually one or at most two fits and rarely going on to demonstrate a state of continued seizures known as *status epilepticus.*

2.2.6.1.3. Psychological State

The withdrawal symptomatology includes moderate to high levels of *anxiety* and a strong drive to obtain the drug. In addition, somewhere between 5% and 15% of individuals develop an OBS and/or a *hallucination/delirium* state. With the barbiturates, probably at least one-half of people showing convulsions during withdrawal go on to a delirium if not treated.[3]

2.2.6.1.4. Relevant Laboratory Tests

Because the CNS withdrawal syndrome is potentially more severe than any other type of drug withdrawal, it is essential that an adequate physical exmaination be carried out and all baseline laboratory tests (including most of the chemistries and blood counts listed in Table 1.5) be considered. A toxicologic screen (10 cc blood or 50 cc urine) may or may not reveal evidence of the drug, depending upon the length of time since the last drug dose and the specific substance involved. It is imperative that the physical condition be carefully monitored throughout the acute withdrawal syndrome.

2.2.6.2. Treatment (See Section 6.2.6.2.)

The treatment of depressant withdrawal follows a relatively simple paradigm, consisting of a good *physical evaluation, general supportive care,* and *treatment of the actual withdrawal* itself (including recognition that symptoms have occurred because a depressant drug was stopped too quickly).[2,4,31]

1. Because of the possibility of the development of an OBS or convulsions, it is probably safest to carry out withdrawal in a *hospital setting.*[3]

2. The poor physical condition of many drug abusers necessitates that each patient receive an adequate *physical examination* and general *screening laboratory procedures.*

3. Assuming a good physical evaluation and that good nutrition, rest, and *multivitamins* are being offered the patient, treatment of the *actual withdrawal* itself can begin. The two most usual withdrawal regimens (neither of which is clearly superior) are outlined in Table 2.4. At this point, it is a good idea to develop a *flow sheet* of all symptoms as evaluated every four hours, along with the drug doses given.[4]

    a. The pentobarbital (short-to-intermediate–acting barbiturate) method.[4, 31]

        i. This involves utilizing an *oral test dose of 200 mg* of the drug (usually pentobarbital) and evaluating the individual one to two hours later. If the patient is sleeping at that time, he is probably not addicted to depressant drugs, and no active medication will be needed.[4]

        ii. If, after two hours, the individual is showing severe tremors, orthostatic hypotension, or other signs of withdrawal, it is assumed that severe withdrawal is imminent and an alternate schedule of withdrawal is established, as discussed under number v below.

       iii. If, at two hours, the individual looks normal, it is possible to wait two to five hours and retest with 200 mg of an oral intermediate-acting barbiturate and continue with test doses during the day to establish the final level needed during the first 24 hours.

       iv. In this instance, the barbiturate is then withdrawn by approximately 100 mg each day. If serious withdrawal symptoms recur, withdrawal is proceeding too quickly, and the

Table 2.4
Treatment of Depressant Withdrawal[4, 30-32]

I. Pentobarbital method
    Test dose: 200 mg
            If patient falls asleep, no treatment needed.
            If no reaction, repeat dose Q 2 hours.

    Determine dose for 24 hours. Divide QID.

    Stabilize for 2 days.

    Decrease by 100 mg/day.

II. Phenobarbital method
    Calculate needed dose. Give 30 mg phenobarbital for each 100 mg pentobarbital or equivalent.

    Stabilize for 2 days.

    Give QID.

    Decrease by 30 mg each day.

---

patient should be administered an extra 200-mg dose of the barbiturate IM, he should be restabilized at the needed dose, and withdrawal should be begun once more.

v. For those patients who demonstrate severe signs of withdrawal after the administration of a 200-mg short-to-intermediate–acting barbiturate test dose, Sapira *et al.*[4] recommend that the patient be given 400 mg of oral barbiturates, be reevaluated every two hours, and be carefully titrated in order to determine the probably high dependent dose.

b. The second withdrawal regimen utilizes a *longer-acting barbiturate, phenobarbital* (Luminal), which has a half-life of 12–24 hours.[30] This approach is based on the ease with which stable blood levels of this longer-acting drug can be reached—but suffers the drawback of some difficulty in titrating the original dose accurately.

i. One begins by estimating the dose of the drug abused and giving approximately 32 mg of phenobarbital for each 100 mg of estimated abused barbiturates, each 250 mg of a drug like glutethimide (Doriden), each 400 mg of meprobamate (Equanil), each 5 mg of diazepam (Valium), and each 25 mg of chlordiazepoxide (Librium). The total dose of phenobarbital is divided into portions to be given four times per day, with extra given if the patient begins to demonstrate signs of withdrawal.

ii. One or two doses (or more) are withheld if the patient appears too sleepy or demonstrates some signs of intoxication, such as nystagmus[20] or ataxia.

iii. The required dose is then utilized for two days, given in divided doses at 6 A.M., noon, 6 P.M., and midnight—the largest dose (approximately 1.5 times the other dose) being given at midnight.

iv. After this, the dose is decreased by approximately 30 mg per day—utilizing a 200-mg IM dose if needed to control the emergence of serious withdrawal symptoms.[32] If the patient looks sleepy or confused, the next dose should be withheld until he clears.[20]

In utilizing either regimen, it has not been shown that it is necessary to include diphenylhydantoin (Dilantin).[33] It also must be emphasized that the information presented in Table 2.4 is a rough outline and that the individual dose must be titrated for the specific patient. The goal is to reach a drug level at 24 hours that decreases withdrawal symptomatology without intoxicating the patient or making him overly sleepy. As with any drug that has a half-life of more than a few hours, it is important to recognize that the drug could accumulate in the body over time. This danger is especially important in elderly patients.

2.2.7. Medical Problems

There are few medical disorders known to be unique to depressant abusers. The conditions developed depend on the specific drug taken and the route of administration. A few "special" problems are discussed below.

1. There is much anecdotal information on the ability of these drugs to *decrease memory* over an extended period of time—perhaps even permanently. However, this phenomenon has not been well worked out, although there is a possibility of permanent neurologic damage.[34,35]

2. IV users can be expected to develop any of the problems that can result from contaminated needles. These include hepatitis, tetanus, abscesses, etc., as described in Section 6.2.8., for opiates.

3. A special problem can result from the (usually inadvertent) injection of these drugs into an artery. The resulting painful muscle and nervous tissue necrosis can necessitate amputation of the limb.[36]

REFERENCES

1. Harvey, S. C. Chapter 9: Hypnotics and sedatives. In L. S. Goodman & A. Gilman (Eds.), *The Pharmacological Basis of Therapeutics*. New York: Macmillan, 1975, pp. 102–124.

2. Jaffe, J. H. Chapter 16: Drug addiction and drug abuse. In L. S. Goodman & A. Gilman (Eds.), *The Pharmacological Basis of Therapeutics*. New York: Macmillan, 1975, pp. 284–324.

3. National Clearing House for Drugs Abuse Information. *The CNS Depressant Withdrawal Syndrome and Its Management. An Annotated Bibliography: 1950–1973*. Rockville, Md.: National Institute on Drug Abuse, 1975.

4. Sapira, J. D., & Cherubin, C. E. Drug Abuse. A Guide for the Clinician. *Excerpta Medica, Amsterdam*. New York: American Elsevier, 1975.

5. Covi, L., Lipman, J. H., Pattison, J. H., *et al.* Length of treatment with anxiolytic sedatives and response to their sudden withdrawal. *Acta Psychiatrica Scandinavica.* 49:51–64, 1973.

6. Haskell, D. Withdrawal of diazepam. *Journal of the American Medical Association,* 233(2):134, 1975.

7. Essig, C. F. Newer sedative drugs that can cause states of intoxication and dependence of barbiturate type. *Journal of the American Medical Association. 196*(8):126–129, 1966.

8. Pascarelli, E. F. Methaqualone abuse, the quiet epidemic. *Journal of the American Medical Association. 224*:1512–1514, 1973.

9. Kay, D. C., Blackburn, A. B., Buckingham, J. A., & Karacan, I. Chapter 4: Human pharmacology of sleep. In R. L. Williams & I. Karacan (Eds.), *Pharmacology of Sleep*. New York: Wiley, 1976, pp. 95–210.

10. Kales, A., Bixler, E. O., Tan, T.-L., *et al.* Chronic hypnotic-drug use. Ineffectiveness, drug-withdrawal insomnia, and dependence. *Journal of the American Medical Association,* 227(5):513–518, 1974.

11. Raskind, M. A., & Eisdorfer, C. When elderly patients can't sleep. *Drug Therapy.* August 1977, pp. 44–50.

12. Dement, W. C. *Some must watch while others sleep. The Portable Stanford.* Stanford: Stanford Alumni Association, 1972.

13. Greenblatt, D. J., & Shader, R. I. *Benzodiazepines in Clinical Practice*. New York: Raven Press, 1974.

14. Hubbard, B., & Kripke, D. F. Hypnotic and minor tranquilizer use among inpatients and after discharge. *The International Journal of the Addictions. 11*(3):403–408, 1976.

15. Parry, H. J., Balter, M. B., & Mellinger, G. D. National patterns of psychotherapeutic drug use. *Archives of General Psychiatry. 28*:769–783, 1973.

16. Abrahams, M. J., Armstrong, J., & Whitlock, F. A. Drug dependence in Brisbane. *The Medical Journal of Australia. 2*:397–404, 1970.

17. Ewing, J. A. Diagnosis and management of depressant drug dependence. *American Journal of Psychiatry, 123*:909–917, 1967.

18. Bakewell, W. E., & Wikler, A. Incidence in a university hospital psychiatric ward. *Journal of the American Medical Association. 196*:(8), 1966.

19. Woody, G. E., O'Brien, C. P., & Greenstein, R. Misuse and abuse of diazepam: An increasingly common medical problem. *The International Journal of the Addictions. 10*(5):843–848, 1975.

20. Cohen, S. Valium: Its use and abuse. *Drug Abuse and Alcoholism Newsletter.* San Diego: Vista Hill Foundation, 5(4), May 1976.

21. Brophy, J. J. Suicide attempts with psychotherapeutic drugs. *Archives of General Psychiatry. 17*:652–657, 1967.

22. Diaz, J. Phenobarbital: Effects of long-term administration on behavior and brain of artificially reared rats. *Science. 199*:90–91, 1978.

23. Good, M. I. The concept of drug automatism. *American Journal of Psychiatry. 133*(8):948–952, 1976.

24. Setter, J. G. Emergency treatment of acute barbiturate intoxication. In P. G. Bourne (Ed.), *A Treatment Manual for Acute Drug Abuse Emergencies*. Washington, D.C.: U.S. Government Printing Office, 1974, pp. 49–53.

25. Afifi, A. A., Sacks, S. T., Liu, V. Y., *et al.* Accumulative prognostic index for patients with barbiturate, gluthethimide and meprobamate intoxication. *New England Journal of Medicine. 285*:1497–1502, 1971.

26. Cronin, R. J., Klingler, E. L., Avasthi, S., *et al.* Chapter 3, Part III: The treatment of nonbarbiturate sedative overdosage. In P. G. Bourne (Ed.), *A Treatment Manual for Acute Drug Abuse Emergencies*. Washington, D.C.: U.S. Government Printing Office, 1974, pp. 58–61.

27. Kirshbaum, R. J., & Carollo, V. J. Reversible iso-electric EEG in barbiturate coma. *Journal of the American Medical Association. 212*(7):1215, 1970.

28. Raskind, M., & Eisdorfer, C. Psychopharmacology of the aged. In L. L. Simpson (Ed.), *Drug Treatment of Mental Disorders*. New York: Raven Press, 1976, pp. 237–266.

29. Schuckit, M. A. Geriatric alcoholism and drug abuse. *The Gerontologist. 17*:168, 1977.

30. Wesson, D. R., & Smith, D. E. Managing the barbiturate withdrawal syndrome. In P. G. Bourne (Ed.), *A Treatment Manual for Acute Drug Abuse Emergencies*. Washington, D.C.: U.S. Government Printing Office, 1974, pp. 54–57.

31. Wikler, A. Diagnosis and treatment of drug dependence of the barbiturate type. *American Journal of Psychiatry. 125*(6):758–765, 1968.

32. Smith, D. E., & Wesson, D. R. Phenobarbital technique for treatment of barbiturate dependence. *Archives of General Psychiatry. 24*:56–60, 1971.

33. Medical Letter. *Diagnosis and Management of Reactions to Drug Abuse*. New Rochelle, N.Y.: The Medical Letter, Vol. 19(3), Feb. 1977.

34. Grant, I., & Mohns, L. Chronic cerebral effects of alcohol and drug abuse. *The International Journal of the Addictions. 10*(5):883–920, 1975.

35. Grant, I., & Judd, L. L. Neuropsychological and EEG disturbances in polydrug users. *American Journal of Psychiatry. 133*(9):1039–1042, 1976.

Alcoholism: An Introduction

3.1. INTRODUCTION

3.1.1. General Comments

Alcohol, nicotine, and caffeine are the most widely used drugs in Western civilization, with alcohol the most potent and destructive of the three. Probably reflecting this, there is a great deal of information available on the epidemiology, the natural history, and the treatment of alcohol-related disorders; thus, this drug is used as a prototype for the discussion of other pharmacologic agents. Information on alcohol is presented in two chapters, with Chapter 3 covering the pharmacology of alcohol, definitional problems surrounding this drug, the epidemiology of drinking patterns and problems, the natural history of alcoholism, and some data on etiology. Chapter 4 is an overview of treatment.

3.1.2. Some Definitions

3.1.2.1. General Comments

It is important at this point to note the distinction between studies of *drinking practices* and studies of *alcoholism*. The vast majority of Americans drink, and a substantial minority (one-third or more) of young men drink to the point of getting into transient difficulties.[1] However, these young men usually do not go on to develop the persistent, serious alcohol-related difficulties that might be termed *alcoholism*.

I diagnose to indicate prognosis and select treatment. For this purpose, the entity must be clearly defined by objective criteria that can be utilized by different clinicians in different settings; people with the syndrome must have a somewhat homogeneous, predictable course (seen in follow-up); and the disorder must not represent the prodrome of yet another diagnosis.[2,3] To be used to maximal benefit, the diagnostic criteria should have been applied to individuals randomly assigned to different treatments to determine which is the most effective and the least dangerous approach.

Unfortunately, the *Second Diagnostic Manual of the American Psychiatric Association* (DSM II) does not use objective terms nor demonstrates any predictive validity for the syndromes outlined under alcoholism, with the result that the labels tend to be applied in an inconsistent manner.[4,5] The next edition of the DSM (DSM III) appears to improve upon the situation, presenting a definition for alcoholism requiring life problems as well as evidence of psychological or physical dependence.[6] The prognostic implications of this new definition have not yet been fully established, and, thus, I use the similar (but not identical) problem-oriented approach outlined below. The more limited problems associated with alcohol abuse (e.g., alcoholic hallucinosis, pathological intoxication, etc.) are discussed in Section 4.2.

3.1.2.2. Definition of Alcoholism

To be clinically useful, the diagnostic criteria must be stated in relatively objective terms, avoiding such judgments as "he drinks too much" or "I *feel* that he is becoming too psychologically dependent." There is no one best definition for alcoholism, and the different criteria overlap a great deal.

1. The *quantity–frequency–variability* (QFV)[7] approach attempts to gather accurate information on drinking patterns and then to place an individual in a "deviant" category when the alcohol intake differs statistically from the average. While this scheme has great relevance to studies of drinking practices, its usefulness is limited by the difficulty in obtaining good information about alcohol intake because of the reticence of the individual to admit his pattern and his decreased memory at rapidly rising blood-alcohol levels.[8]

2. The second rubric, *psychological dependence,* is based on the occurrence of a series of subjective experiences relating drinking to such problems as stockpiling liquor, taking drinks before going to a party, and otherwise demonstrating that the individual is psychologically uncomfortable unless there is alcohol around.[9] It is very difficult, if not impossible, to quantify this approach objectively.

3. A third diagnostic scheme, fairly widely used by physicians, centers on the occurrence of *withdrawal* or *abstinence* symptoms when an individual stops taking alcohol.[10] However, between 85% and 95% of people experiencing withdrawal have only the more minor symptoms.[11] In this mild form, it can be difficult to distinguish withdrawal from a

hangover or a case of the flu. In any event, this definition is restrictive, as many individuals who have serious life-impairment and medical problems and who may suffer an alcohol-related death have never demonstrated obvious signs of physiological withdrawal.

4. The definition that probably has the greatest usefulness to clinicians centers on the occurrence of serious social or health *problems related to alcohol*.[2,12,13] The research criteria note the occurrence of any major life problem related to alcohol, including a marital separation or divorce, or multiple arrests, or physical evidence that alcohol has harmed health (e.g., a cardiomyopathy, cirrhosis, etc.), or loss of a job or layoff related to drinking.[14]

As is true with any clinical diagnosis, the criteria can be "bent" for an individual who comes close but does not quite fit the research definition and is thus labeled a "probable" alcoholic. In this circumstance, the patient may receive the same general treatment as the definite alcoholic, but I constantly recheck my diagnosis and recognize the lowered level of certainty in predicting the future course.

3.1.2.3. Primary versus Secondary Alcoholism (See Figure 3.1.)

To use diagnosis for prognosis and selection of treatment, it is important that one look separately at those cases that *might* be a complication of

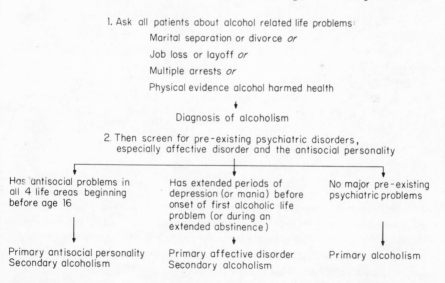

Figure 3.1. The diagnosis of alcoholism. From Schuckit, M. A. Treatment of alcoholism in office and outpatient settings. In J. H. Mendelson & N. K. Mello (Eds.), *Diagnosis and Treatment of Alcoholism*. New York: McGraw-Hill, copyright © 1979. Reprinted with permission of McGraw-Hill Book Company.

another disorder (secondary) and those that are more straightforward alcoholism (primary). The paradigm is similar to that used for patients with pneumonia: one case might be related to an immune deficiency; another pneumonitis might be secondary to trauma; yet another might reflect the consequences of congestive heart failure. Each exemplifies *secondary* pneumonia, where the prognosis and the major treatment efforts are dictated by the primary illness (e.g., the trauma or the heart failure).

In a similar manner, a patient who develops his alcohol abuse after the onset of another major psychiatric disorder has *secondary alcoholism*, while one who shows no evidence of a preexisting major psychiatric problem would be labeled a *primary alcoholic*.[13,15] It is the primary alcoholics who can be thought of as having the "disease" alcoholism and who are most likely to fit the natural history outlined below.

Secondary alcoholism can occur in the midst of almost any psychiatric picture, but it is most likely to be seen with the antisocial personality and in individuals with primary affective disorder. The remaining personality syndromes noted in the DSM II are not stated clearly enough to be clinically useful here.

3.1.2.3.1. Primary Antisocial Personality with Secondary Alcoholism

The antisocial personality or sociopath can be defined as an individual who demonstrates antisocial life problems in *all four* life areas of family, school, police, and peers, beginning prior to age 16 and prior to the onset of alcohol and drug abuse.[2,13,16] The sociopath runs a course of serious violence and criminal behavior, thus carrying a prognosis different from that of the primary alcoholic. Evaluations of both public and private inpatient alcoholic programs indicate that approximately 20% of male alcoholics and 5% of female alcoholics have primary antisocial personalities with secondary alcoholism.[13,17]

3.1.2.3.2. Primary Affective Disorder with Secondary Alcoholism

Disorders of mood, or affect, can entail either a serious depression or an episode of euphoria, hyperirritability, grandiosity, and disorganized thinking that is termed *mania*.[2] Because most people with primary affective disorder have depressions only (unipolar affective disorder), the major discussion here will center on depression, not mania.

When an episode of sadness that represents a change from the person's normal level of functioning persists for at least two weeks, occurs all day every day, and is accompanied by changes in body functioning (e.g., insomnia, lethargy, constipation, etc.) and changes in mind functioning (e.g., inability to concentrate, the future looking hopeless, loss of interest in usual activities, etc.), the diagnosis of depressive disorder can be made. This episode of sadness is quite different from the normally transient grief reaction or other despondencies accompanying a loss. When the depressive episode occurs in the absence of preexisting psychiatric disorders, including alcoholism, the label of *primary affective disorder* can be assigned, with its implications for prognosis and treatment.[2]

Studies of inpatient alcoholics have shown that about 20% of women and 5% of men meeting the criteria for alcoholism have had affective disorder episodes either *prior to* their first major alcoholic life problem or during a period of three or more months when they were not actively drinking.[13,15,17] Such individuals would be labeled *primary affective disorder* and *secondary alcoholics*.

3.1.2.3.3. Other Diagnoses

When careful diagnostic criteria are used,[2] alcoholism is rarely secondary to disorders other than the antisocial personality or primary affective disorder. Less than 5% of alcoholics demonstrate schizophrenia (the very slow onset of social withdrawal, hallucinations, and/or delusions that are persistent and seen during an extended abstinence[2]) or other psychiatric disorders such as hysteria (Briquet's disease) and anxiety neurosis. The confusion in the literature on the relationship between alcoholism and schizophrenia[18] occurs when investigators use loose criteria for schizophrenia whereby relatively benign or transient paranoid or hallucinatory psychoses, which may accompany heavy use of alcohol (see Section 4.2.4.), are mislabeled as schizophrenia.

The key to accurate labeling is in taking a very careful history of the chronology of the development of psychiatric symptoms from both the patient and a resource person such as the spouse. Primary sociopathy is easily distinguished from primary alcoholism through gathering information on the extent of antisocial problems occurring before age 16. Primary affective disorder is more difficult to establish because alcohol causes serious depression.[15,19] Thus, only depressions or manias occurring before the first major life problem related to alcohol or episodes occurring during an extended period of abstinence qualify as primary affective disorder and secondary alcoholism. The primary schizophrenic should demonstrate persistent and serious social withdrawal and hallucinations/delusions that have occurred before the onset of serious alcohol problems and remain throughout extended periods of abstinence.

3.2. PHARMACOLOGY OF ALCOHOL

3.2.1. General Comments

This widely used drug is a central nervous system (CNS) depressant that, in high enough doses, is an anesthetic. It adversely affects almost all body systems, interfering with either cell membrane functioning, intracellular respiration, or energy processing in most body cells, especially those in the CNS.[20-22] While the primary action of alcohol on the CNS is depression, at lower doses behavioral stimulant properties predominate, a fact that may be related to a direct stimulant effect of alcohol or a differential depression of inhibitory neurons at relatively low blood-alcohol concentrations.[23] The CNS depression occurs at all levels of the brain, with the first noted actions occurring in the reticular activating system and those areas most closely involved with complex functions—the cortex.[23]

The final level of behavioral impairment depends upon the person's age, weight, sex, and prior experience with alcohol, as well as his level of tolerance. Table 3.1 gives a rough outline of what can be expected in a nontolerant individual, with results ranging from minor impairment in motor coordination, sensation, and mood at low doses to amnesia and Stage 1 anesthesia for blood levels exceeding 300 mg of alcohol per 100 ml of blood (mg %). Doses of 400–700 mg % can cause coma, respiratory failure, and death,[21] although tolerant individuals may be awake and able to talk at blood levels exceeding 780 mg %.[24] Note that 100 mg % is equivalent to 0.1 gram/100 ml.[25]

Table 3.1
Rough Correlation between Blood-Alcohol Level
and Behavioral/Motor Impairment[21]

Rising blood alcohol level in mg/100 ml blood (mg%)	Expected effect
20–99	Impaired coordination, euphoric
100–199	Ataxia, decreased mentation, poor judgment, labile mood
200–299	Marked ataxia and slurred speech, poor judgment, labile mood, nausea and vomiting
300–399	Stage I Anesthesia, memory lapse, labile mood
400 and above	Respiratory failure, coma, death

3.2.2. Effects on the Body

When alcohol is taken in moderation by an individual in good health, the pathological changes appear to be totally reversible, but at higher doses or in individuals who are ill, damage to various body systems can be life-threatening. Because the physiological toxicity of alcohol has been reviewed in depth in other texts,[20,21,26,27] a very brief review is given here.

1. In the *digestive system*, alcohol is associated with high rates of cancers of all levels of the digestive tract, especially the esophagus and stomach[28]; high rates of ulcer disease[29]; and elevated rates of inflammation of the stomach (gastritis), or pancreas (pancreatitis), fatty liver, alcoholic hepatitis, and cirrhosis.[30] Even at low doses, alcohol disturbs the ability of the liver to produce sugar (gluconeogenesis) and shunts building blocks into the production of fats.[22]

2. In the *neurologic system*, the chronic intake of alcohol results in deterioration of both peripheral nerves to the hands and feet (a peripheral neuropathy seen in 5–15% of alcoholics)[31] and temporary as well as permanent organic brain syndromes associated with both the direct effect of alcohol and specific vitamin deficiencies, such as the thiamine-related Wernicke–Korsakoff syndrome[32] (seen in less than 5% of alcoholics). It has been estimated that between 15% and 30% of nursing-home patients with organic brain syndromes are alcoholics whose alcohol-induced organicity has become permanent.[33] Additional problems associated with the CNS involve a rapidly developing permanent uncoordination (cerebellar degeneration), which is seen in less that 1% of alcohlics[34] and other more dramatic but even rarer neurologic disorders that can result in rapid death.[31]

3. It has also been estimated that one-quarter of alcoholics develop diseases of the heart or *cardiovascular system*,[35] as alcohol, a striated muscle toxin, produces a heart inflammation or myocardiopathy and hypertention and elevates blood fats, including cholesterol.[20,21,35] In addition, alcohol in doses as low as one drink can decrease the cardiac output of blood in nonalcoholics with heart disease and diminish the warning signs of pain while increasing the potential heart damage or ischemia in patients with angina.[36]

4. Alcohol also decreases the production of all types of *blood cells*, with resulting large red blood cell anemia (a macrocytosis, probably related to folic acid deficiency), decreased production and efficiency of white cells (probably leading to an increased predisposition toward infection), and decreased production of clotting factors and platelets (probably related to increased bruising and gastrointestinal bleeding[35,37–39]). There is also a decrease in thymus-derived lymphocytes, which might relate to the increased rates of cancers seen in alcoholics.[40]

5. *Body muscle* is also sensitive to alcohol, and an alcoholic binge can result in muscle inflammation or, in chronic abusers, muscle wasting, primarily in the shoulders and hips.[30]

6. Through a variety of mechanisms, alcohol induces a number of other *blood test* abnormalities, including those of liver function, glucose, blood components, creatinine phosphokinase (CPK), and uric acid.[41]

3.2.3. Effects on Mental Processes

In addition to the physiological changes that occur with alcohol, there are a number of important emotional consequences. With modest intake, at peak or decreasing blood-alcohol levels, most people (alcoholics and "normals") experience sadness, anxiety, irritability, insomnia, decreased sexual potency (for males), and a whole host of resulting interpersonal problems.[15,19,42] At persistent higher doses, alcohol can cause almost any psychiatric symptom,[38] including temporary pictures of intense sadness, auditory hallucinations and/or paranoia in the presence of clear thought processes (a clear sensorium),[43] and intense anxiety.[39]

3.2.4. Alcohol Metabolism

Alcohol is fully absorbed from the lining or membranes of the digestive tract, especially in the stomach and the proximal portion of the small intestine. Only 5–15% is excreted directly through the lungs, sweat, and urine, with the remainder being metabolized in the liver at a rate of approximately one drink per hour, the equivalent of 7 g of ethanol per hour, with 1 g equaling 1 ml of 100% alcohol.[21] The usual route of metabolism is via the enzyme alcohol dehydrogenase, although some additional alcohol is metabolized in the liver microsomal system, as shown in Figure 3.2. Thus, the major product of alcohol metabolism is acetaldehyde, a very toxic substance that, fortunately, is quickly metabolized to carbon dioxide and water through a variety of mechanisms.

3.2.5. Tolerance and Physical Dependence

Toleration of higher doses of ethanol occurs rapidly and parallels what has already been discussed about the depressants in Section 2.1.1.3. This tolerance is both metabolic, primarily through a slight increase in the liver microsomal ethanol oxidizing system (MEOS), and pharmacodynamic, the apparent result of direct adaptation of CNS tissues to alcohol.[44] Cross-tolerance to other CNS-depressing drugs occurs, but it must be remembered that concomitant administration of two or more CNS depressants may potentiate the effects of both.

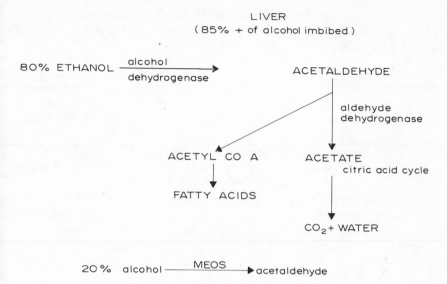

Figure 3.2. The metabolism of alcohol.[21,22]

Alcohol also produces a level of physical addiction that results in a withdrawal syndrome almost identical to that described for the depressants.[45] This is discussed in Section 4.2.6.

3.3. EPIDEMIOLOGY OF DRINKING AND ALCOHOLISM

Most people drink, and many have minor problems, but few demonstrate a lifestyle centered around alcohol (i.e., alcoholism).

3.3.1. Drinking Patterns

Over two-thirds of American men drink more than just occasionally, with a male to female ratio of approximately 1.3 to 1.[46] The peak years, with highest percentages of drinkers and greatest per capita consumption, are probably between 16 and 25, with a decrease with age. At any stage of life, the chances of being a *drinker* (not an alcoholic) are higher for people with higher levels of education, higher socioeconomic status, and Italian or Jewish heritage.[46,47]

The average adult consumes 2.7 gallons of absolute alcohol per year, with a resultant total expenditure of many billions per year in the United States—representing almost 3% of total personal expenditures.[47] Between a quarter and a half of young men experience transient alcohol-related problems, such as arguments with friends, missing time from work, or a drunk-driving arrest.[1] These problems alone do not predict future alcoholism, and most individuals drift away from these problems with increasing age.[1,48]

3.3.2. Alcoholism

Utilizing a rigorous criterion for alcoholism centering on serious life problems (see Section 3.1.2.), it has been estimated that between 5% and 10% of the adult male population in the United States will demonstrate alcoholism at some time during their lives.[47,49] Because of the high level of physical pathology associated with heavy drinking, 20–35% of male general medical or surgical patients are alcoholic.[47]

The highest rates of *alcoholism* are seen in men aged 30–50 years, with rates increasing with lower socioeconomic strata, lower income and education, and among Catholics—especially French and Irish.[47] However, it is important to recognize that alcoholism is a problem of all socioeconomic strata, all ages, all religions, all parts of the country, and both sexes.

3.4. NATURAL HISTORY OF ALCOHOLISM

3.4.1. General Comments (See Figure 3.3.)

Once the diagnosis of primary alcoholism has been carefully established, it is possible to estimate the prognosis or natural course of the disorder. The average primary alcoholic, male or female, demonstrates the first major alcohol-related life problem in the late 20s to early 30s,[50] with most alcoholics presenting for treatment in their early 40s—after more than a decade of difficulties.[51] If alcohol problems continue, the

1. Usual age of onset   28-33
   First major problem

2. Usual age entering treatment   40

3. Usual age of death   55-60
   Leading causes: heart disease
                          cancer
                          accidents
                          suicide

4. In any year, abstinence alternates with active drinking

5. "Spontaneous remission" rate *or*
   Response to nonspecific intervention   1/10-1/3

Figure 3.3. The natural history of primary alcoholism. From Schuckit, M. A. Treatment of alcoholism in office and outpatient settings. In J. H. Mendelson & N. K. Mello (Eds.), *Diagnosis and Treatment of Alcoholism*. New York: McGraw-Hill, copyright © 1979. Reprinted with permission of McGraw-Hill Book Company.

alcoholic is likely to die 15 years earlier than the general population,[26,27] with the leading causes of death (in approximately decreasing order of importance) being heart disease, cancer, accidents, and suicide. These leading death causes do not include the series of disorders found at markedly higher rates in alcoholics than in the general population, such as cirrhosis, pancreatitis, infections, etc.

The course of alcoholism is a fluctuating one, with very few, if any, alcoholics staying persistently drunk until they die. The usual alcohlic is a blue-collar or white-collar worker who alternates periods of abstinence (and times when he is drinking very little) with periods of serious alcohol misuse. In any given month, one-half of alcohlics will be abstinent, with a mean of four months of being dry in any one-year to two-year period.[52] Thus, the average alcoholic has spontaneous periods of abstinence and marked decreases in drinking, which appear to alternate with heavy drinking times.

Alcoholism is not a hopeless disorder. Not only can one expect improvement with treatment, but there is good reason to estimate that as high as one-third of alcoholics learn to abstain or to seriously limit their drinking without any exposure to a formal treatment regimen.[38,39,53,54] The chance of demonstrating spontaneous remission probably increases with the same factors that indicate a good prognosis for those entering treatment (e.g., having a job, living with a family, having no police record, etc.).

3.5. ETIOLOGY

As noted in Chapter 1, a clinically oriented handbook has little room to discuss etiologic theories in great depth. I turn to this topic now to demonstrate both how difficult etiology is to study and how people tend to state erroneously tentative hypotheses as proven fact. As we shall see, a theory that makes sense is not necessarily true, and the demonstration that Factor A is related to Factor B does not mean that the former caused the latter.

3.5.1. Psychological Theories

These usually involve comparisons of alcoholics and nonalcoholics on performance on psychological tests. The approach at times neglects the possibility that the psychological attributes of alcoholics who have been drinking heavily for 10 years may be the consequence of their lifestyle rather than the original cause. Proponents of psychological theories may also fail to differentiate between studies of why people drink and why people become alcoholic.

These theories have included the "tension-reduction hypothesis," which (despite the fact that the majority of physiological evidence indicates that alcohol increases tension) states that alcoholics drink in an attempt to decrease their levels of stress.[55] A second set of important theories centers on the premise that people begin to drink, drink abusively, or remain alcoholic because alcohol, in some way, reinforces or rewards their behavior through inducing pleasure, removing discomfort, enhancing social interactions, and fulfilling the need to feel powerful or, on the other hand, helping them to self-destruct or abolish unpleasant memories.[52]

3.5.2. Sociocultural Theories

A second approach centers on sociocultural theories, utilizing observations of similarities and differences between cultural groups and subgroups as they relate to drinking practices.[56] The major importance of this approach is heuristic, and no factors that are purported to be important in the development of alcoholism in one culture have been shown to generalize to most other cultures. An example would be the statements that Jews and Italians have low rates of alcoholism *because* children are introduced to alcohol within the home setting and alcohol is used as part of religious ceremonies—a theory that ignores the very high rate of alcoholism among the French, for whom both factors also operate.[55]

3.5.3. Biological Theories

A series of biological theories is found in the literature, including the possibility that alcoholics are seeking relief from an innate hypoglycemia, that they have allergies to alcohol or the congeners found in alcoholic beverages, or that a differential brain responsiveness to alcohol exists in alcoholics.[55] Once again, it has not been established whether the physiological abnormalities of alcoholics were the initial cause of the heavy drinking or resulted from a lifestyle of relatively poor nutrition, high stress, and high doses of ethanol.

One theory, which has had a great impact in the field by developing a focus on the chemical changes in nervous-system functioning that result from alcohol, is the possibility that alcohol may produce a morphinelike substance in the brains of certain individuals that may subsequently be responsible for the level of addiction.[57]

3.5.4. Genetic Factors

A series of studies has established the probable importance of genetic factors in the genesis of primary alcoholism. This disorder has been shown to run strongly within *families,* and the rate of concordance (or sameness) for alcoholism in identical *twins* is much higher than in nonidentical twins or same-sex siblings. A number of potential genetic *markers* (such as blood types) have been found to associate with alcoholism, and some biologic factors that influence the patterns of alcohol consumption in animals have been identified.[55] The most important information, however, comes from *separation* or adoption-type studies done in both the United States and Denmark, demonstrating that the children of alcoholic biologic parents separated from their parents early in life and raised without knowledge of their natural parents have markedly elevated rates of alcoholism, while the children of nonalcoholics adopted into the homes of alcoholics do not show elevated rates of alcohol problems as adults.[58]

Thus the best data to date indicate that alcoholism is a genetically influenced disorder with a rate of heritability (i.e., the chance of inheriting the disorder) similar to that expected for diabetes or peptic ulcer disease. This finding may have great importance in helping to elucidate the psychological, social, and cultural factors impacting on the genesis of alcoholism. It may now be possible to study prospectively groups of individuals at high risk for alcoholism and to identify those factors that determine whether the predisposition is expressed and to identify other causative factors.

REFERENCES

1. Cahalan, D. *Problem Drinkers.* San Francisco: Jossey-Bass, 1970.
2. Woodruff, R. A., Goodwin, D. W., & Guze, S. B. *Psychiatric Diagnosis.* New York: Oxford University Press, 1974.
3. Guze, S. B. The need for toughmindedness in psychiatric thinking. *Southern Medical Journal.* 63:662–671, 1970.
4. *Diagnostic and Statistical Manual of Mental Disorders* (II). Washington, D.C.: American Psychiatric Association, 1968.
5. Schuckit, M., & Gunderson, E. K. E. The use of alcoholic subtype diagnoses in the U.S. Navy. *Diseases of the Nervous System.* 35:231–236, 1974.
6. The Task Force on Nomenclature and Statistics of the American Psychiatric Association. *Diagnostic and Statistical Manual of Mental Disorders.* Washington, D.C.: American Psychiatric Association, 1978.
7. Cahalan, D. A multivariate analysis of correlates of drinking-related problems in a community study. *Social Problems.* 17:234–247, 1969.
8. Goodwin, D. W., et al. Loss of short term memory as a predictor of the alcoholic blackout. *Nature.* 227:201, 1970.
9. Barry, H., III. Personality and the alcoholic: Personality of the individual vulnerable to alcoholism and associated characteristics. In N. Kessel, A. Hawker, & H. Chalke (Eds.), *Alcoholism: A Medical Profile.* London: B. Edsall, 1974, pp. 43–51.
10. Sellers, E. M., & Kalant, H. Alcohol intoxication and withdrawal. *New England Journal of Medicine,* 294:757–762, 1976.

11. Victor, M. Treatment of alcoholic intoxication and the withdrawal syndrome. *Psychosomatic Medicine. 28:*636–649, 1966.
12. Criteria Committee, National Council of Alcoholism. Criteria for the diagnosis of alcoholism. *American Journal of Psychiatry. 129*(2):127–135, 1972.
13. Schuckit, M. A. Alcoholism and sociopathy: Diagnostic confusion. *Quarterly Journal of Studies on Alcoholism. 34:*157–164, 1973.
14. Schuckit, M. A., Pitts, F. N., Reich, T., *et al.*, Alcoholism. I. Two types of alcoholism in women. *Archives of General Psychiatry. 20:*301–306, 1969.
15. Schuckit, M. A. Depression and alcoholism in women. In M. E. Chafetz (Ed.), Proceedings of the First Annual Alcoholism Conference of the National Institute on Alcohol Abuse and Alcoholism. Washington, D.C.: U. S. Government Printing Office, 1974, pp. 355–363.
16. Robins, L. N. *Deviant Children Grown Up.* Baltimore: Williams & Wilkins, 1966.
17. Schuckit, M. A., & Winokur, G. A short-term follow-up of women alcoholics. *Diseases of the Nervous System. 33:*672–678, 1972.
18. Schuckit, M. A., & Winokur, G. Alcoholic hallucinosis and schizophrenia: A negative study. *The British Journal of Psychiatry. 199*(552):549–550, 1971.
19. Gibson, S., & Becker, J. Changes in alcoholics' self-reported depression. *Quarterly Journal of Studies on Alcohol. 34:*829–836, 1973.
20. Kissin, B., & Begleiter, H. (Eds.). *The Biology of Alcoholism. Vol. 1: Biochemistry.* New York: Plenum Press, 1971.
21. Becker, C.E. *Alcohol as a Drug: A Curriculum on Pharmacology, Neurology and Toxicology.* Baltimore: Williams & Wilkins, 1974.
22. Lieber, C. S. Liver adaptation and injury in alcoholism. *New England Journal of Medicine. 288:*356–362, 1973.
23. Ritchie, J. M. The aliphatic alcohols. In L. S. Goodman & A. Gilman (Eds.), *The Pharmacological Basis of Therapeutics.* New York: Macmillan, 1975, pp. 380–391.
24. Hammond, K. B., Rumack, B. H., & Rodgerson, D. O. Blood ethanol. A report of unusually high levels in a living patient. *Journal of American Medical Association. 226*(1):63–64, 1973.
25. Turner, T. B., Mezey, E., & Kimball, A. W. Measurement of alcohol-related effects in man: Chronic effects in relation to levels of alcohol consumption. Part A. *The Johns Hopkins Medical Journal. 141:*235–248, 1977.
26. Sundby, P. *Alcoholism and Mortality.* Oslo: Universiets-forlaget, 1967.
27. Schmidt, W., & De Lint, J. Causes of death in alcoholics. *Quarterly Journal of Studies on Alcohol. 33:*171–185, 1972.
28. Hakulinen, T., Lehtimak, L., Lentonen, M., *et al.* Cancer morbidity among two male cohorts. *Journal of the National Cancer Institute. 52:*1711–1717, 1974.
29. Lieber, C. S. Alcohol and malnutrition in the pathogenesis of liver disease. *Journal of the American Medical Association. 233:*1077–1082, 1975.
30. Bourne, P. G., & Fox, R. *Alcoholism. Progress in Research and Treatment.* New York: Academic Press, 1973.
31. Fruend, G. Diseases of the nervous system associated with alcoholism. In R. E. Tarter & A. A. Sugerman (Eds.), *Alcoholism: Interdisciplinary Approaches to an Enduring Problem.* Reading, Pa.:Addison-Wesley, 1976.
32. Victor, M., Adams, R. D., & Collins, G. H. *The Wernicke–Korsakoff Syndrome: A Clinical and Pathological Study of 245 Patients, 82 with Post-Mortem Examinations.* Philadelphia: Davis, 1971.

33. Schuckit, M. A., & Miller, P. L. Alcoholism in elderly men: A survey of a general medical ward. *Annals of the New York Academy of Sciences. 273:*558–571, 1976.

34. Kissin, B., & Begleiter, H. (Eds.). *The Biology of Alcoholism. Vol. 3: Clinical Pathology.* New York: Plenum Press, 1971.

35. Wu, C. F., Sudhakar, M., Jaferi, G., et al. Preclinical cardiomyopathy in chronic alcoholics: A sex difference. *American Heart Journal. 91:*281–286, 1971.

36. Horwitz, L. D. Alcohol and heart disease. *Journal of the American Medical Association. 232:*959–960, 1975.

37. Lieber, C. S. (Ed.). *Metabolic Aspects of Alcoholism.* Baltimore: University Park Press, 1977.

38. Schuckit, M. A. Treatment of alcoholism in office and outpatient settings. In J. H. Mendelson & N. K. (Mello (Eds.), *Diagnosis and Treatment of Alcoholism.* New York: McGraw-Hill, 1979, Chapter 6.

39. Schuckit, M. Inpatient and residential approaches to the treatment of alcoholism. In J. H. Mendelson & N. K. Mello (Eds.), *Diagnosis and Treatment of Alcoholism.* New York: McGraw-Hill, 1979, Chapter 7.

40. Lowry, W. S. Alcoholism in cancer of the head and neck. *Laryngoscope. 85:*1275–1280, 1975.

41. Seixas, F. A. Alcohol and its drug interactions. *Annals of Internal Medicine. 83:*86–92, 1975.

42. Tamerin, J. S., & Mendelson, J. Alcoholics' expectancies and recall of experiences and recall of experiences during intoxication. *American Journal of Psychiatry. 126:*1697–1704, 1970.

43. Victor, M., & Hope, J. M. The phenomenon of auditory hallucinations in chronic alcoholism. *Archives of General Psychiatry. 126:*451–481, 1955.

44. Jaffe, J. H. Drug addiction and drug abuse. In L. S. Goodman & A. Gilman (Eds.), *The Pharmacological Basis of Therapeutics.* New York: Macmillan, 1975, pp. 293–324.

45. Kissin, B., & Begleiter, H. (Eds.). *The Biology of Alcoholism. Vol. 2: Physiology and Behavior.* New York: Plenum Press, 1971.

46. Cahalan, D., & Cisin, I. H. American drinking practices: Summary of findings from a national probability sample. I. Extent of drinking by population subgroups. *Quarterly Journal of Studies on Alcohol. 29:*130–152, 1968.

47. Haglund, R. M. J., & Schuckit, M. A. The epidemiology of alcoholism. In N. Estes & E. Heinemann (Eds.), *Alcoholism: Development, Consequences and Interventions.* St. Louis: Mosby, 1977.

48. Fillmore, K. M. Relationships between specific drinking problems in early adulthood and middle age. *Journal of Studies on Alcohol. 36:*882–907, 1975.

49. Schuckit, M. A., & Morrissey, E. R. Alcoholism in women: Some clinical and social perspectives with an emphasis on possible subtypes. In M. Greenblatt & M. A. Schuckit (Eds.), *Alcohol Problems in Women and Children.* New York: Grune & Stratton, 1976.

50. Schuckit, M. A., Rimmer, J., Reich, T., et al. Alcoholism: Antisocial traits in male alcoholics. *British Journal of Psychiatry. 117:*575–576, 1970.

51. Schuckit, M. A. Alcoholism: Natural history and outcome studies. Presented at the Society for Epidemiologic Research Annual Meeting, Seattle, Washington, D.C., June 1977.

52. Ludwig, A. M. On and off the wagon. *Quarterly Journal of Studies on Alcohol. 33:*91–96, 1972.

53. Drew, L. R. H. Alcoholism as a self-limiting disease. *Quarterly Journal of Studies on Alcohol. 29:*956–967, 1968.

54. Smart, R. G. Spontaneous recovery in alcoholics: A review and analysis of the available research. *Drug and Alcohol Dependency*. 1:227–285, 1976.

55. Schuckit, M. A., & Haglund, R. M. J. An overview of the etiologic theories on alcoholism. In N. Estes & E. Heinemann (Eds.), *Alcoholism: Development, Consequences and Interventions*. St. Louis: Mosby, 1977.

56. Roebuck, J. B., & Kessler, R. G. *The Etiology of Alcoholism*. Springfield, Ill.: Charles C Thomas, 1972.

57. Nichols, J. Alcoholism and opiate addiction: Theory and evidence for a genetic link between the two. In O. Forsander & K. Eriksson (Eds.), *Biological Aspects of Alcohol Consumption*. Helsinki, Finland: The Finnish Foundation for Alcohol Studies. 1971.

58. Goodwin, D. *Is Alcoholism Hereditary?* New York: Oxford University Press, 1976.

The Treatment of Alcoholism

4.1. INTRODUCTION

Alcohol is the most commonly abused substance, creating serious medical and psychological problems. I will present an overview of *emergency problems* here, but the extensive discussion of rehabilitation that serves as a prototype for the rehabilitation of substance abusers in general is presented in Chapter 13.

4.1.1. Identification of the Alcoholic

The "obvious" alcoholic who calls in the middle of the night drunk or who has signs of cirrhosis represents a minority of individuals with alcoholism. The usual alcohol-dependent patient is a middle-class family man or homemaker presenting with complaints of insomnia, sadness, nervousness, or interpersonal problems. Because 5–10% of adult men develop alcoholism (the rate for women being approximately one-third of that) and the rate of alcohol problems in medical and surgical inpatients may be over 25%, it is important to consider alcoholism a part of the differential diagnosis for every individual. The index of suspicion should be even higher for those with some of the more typical medical problems, including high blood pressure, ulcer disease, elevated uric acid, a macrocytosis, or any fluctuating medical condition that is otherwise difficult to explain (see Section 3.2.2.).

Therefore, I take the two or three minutes necessary to query *each* patient about alcohol-related life problems. I begin by asking about general areas of difficulty, including: "How are things going with your spouse?" "Have you had any accidents since I last saw you?" "How are things going on the job?" "Have you had any arrests or traffic tickets?" etc. If there is a general life problem, I then try to determine what role, if any, alcohol may have played in that problem and go on to questions about the quantity and frequency of drinking. If the patients appears evasive or if I have any further doubts, I privately interview the spouse.

4.1.2. Obtaining a History

Once I have established either a definitive or a probable diagnosis of alcoholism, I must determine whether or not there are any preexisting primary psychiatric disorders (as outlined in Figure 3.1). Thus, I first do a brief review of antisocial problems early in life, including such questions as "How did you do in school?" "What was the highest grade you completed?" "Did you ever run away from home overnight before you were 16?" "Did you have any police record prior to age 16?" "When you were in junior high school or high school, did you get in a lot of fights and did you ever use a weapon in a fight?" etc. Next, I ask about any depression that occurred daily, all day, for periods of at least two weeks or that was associated with the body and mind changes described in Section 3.1.2.3. If these have occurred, I then determine whether they existed prior to the first major alcohol-related life problem or occurred during a time when the individual had been abstinent for at least three months.

These steps are well worth my time, as complex and perplexing medical and psychological problems associated with alcoholism can be very confusing and can lead to serious complications through improper diagnosis and treatment. I can practice good preventive medicine and save myself a number of middle-of-the-night calls into the emergency room by maintaining a high level of suspicion for alcoholism.

4.2. EMERGENCY SITUATIONS

The most frequent emergency situations for alcoholics involve toxic reactions and accidents. Almost 8% of all emergency room patients have alcohol problems as part of their mode of presentation, rates that increase to 25% for accident victims.[1] Recognition of the presence of alcohol (whether alcoholism is involved or not) is important, as this drug alters the patient's reactions to emergency procedures.

4.2.1. Panic Reaction (See Section 1.6.1.)

4.2.1.1. The Clinical Picture

Alcohol is a depressant drug and thus is rarely involved in acute panics. One possible exception, based on the increased level of anxiety that can be seen during alcohol imbibition as well as during withdrawal, is the induction of acute anxiety attacks characterized by nervousness, hyperventilation, and palpitations.

4.2.1.2. Treatment

After taking an EKG, doing a physical examination, and evaluating to be sure that acute withdrawal is not likely, the cornerstone of treatment is reassurance and education. Of course, I will probably refer these patients for alcohol counseling.

4.2.2. Flashbacks

Flashbacks are not noted with alcohol.

4.2.3. Toxic Reactions (See Sections 1.6.3., 2.2.3., 6.2.3., and 12.4.)

Toxic reactions to alcohol are usually the result of the narrow range between the anesthetic and the lethal doses of this drug or reflect the potentiating interaction seen between alcohol and other CNS depressants (see Section 11.2.3.).

4.2.3.1. The Clinical Picture

The overdose from alcohol results from CNS depression to the point of respiratory and circulatory failure. The danger is heightened when alcohol is taken in combination with other CNS-depressing drugs, such as any of the hypnotics or antianxiety drugs; but can also occur with drugs of other classes, such as the opiates. The clinical picture of an ethanol overdose is basically similar to what has been described for the depressants in Section 2.2.3.

4.2.3.1.1. The History

The patient usually presents smelling of alcohol with a history of a recent ingestion of high doses of alcohol, perhaps accompanied by other CNS depressants, such as sleeping pills (e.g., the barbiturates or flurazepam [Dalmane]) or the antianxiety drugs (e.g., chlordiazepoxide [Librium] or diazepam [Valium]). If no history can be obtained directly from the patient, a friend or relative might supply the relevant information, or there may be obvious evidence of drug ingestion (e.g., empty bottles).

4.2.3.1.2. Physical Signs and Symptoms

These are identical to the physical manifestations reported for other CNS depressants in Section 2.2.3. Basically the patient presents with depressed functioning of the CNS and slowed vital signs, including a slow pulse, a lowered respiratory rate, and a low blood pressure.

4.2.3.1.3. Psychological State

This also resembles the picture described for the other CNS depressants in Section 2.2.3., including signs of severe intoxication (i.e., the person is very drunk) along with confusion and irritability of mood.

4.2.3.1.4. Relevant Laboratory Data

The diagnosis, resting with the history and the physical examination, is aided by the toxicologic screen (10 ml blood or 50 ml urine) for both alcohol and other CNS depressants. The remaining laboratory tests are those necessary to properly exclude other causes of stupor (e.g., low glucose, etc.) and to monitor the physical status (e.g., blood counts and, if the patient is very stuporous, blood gases, as shown in Table 1.5).

4.2.3.2. Treatment

A fatal toxic reaction has been reported with blood alcohol levels as low as 350 mg % in nontolerant individuals.[2] The treatment procedures follow those outlined for CNS depressants in Section 2.2.3.2., but there are a few differences.

1. Treatment involves carrying out the necessary emergency procedures to guarantee adequate ventilation, circulation, and control of shock; a careful evaluation to rule out ancillary medical problems, such as electrolyte disturbances, cardiac disorders, associated infections, subdural hematomas, etc.; and then establishing general supportive measures while the body metabolizes the alcohol.

2. Some investigators report that intravenous fructose slightly increases the rate of ethanol metabolism, but this is not enough to overcome the resulting problems of disturbed sugar metabolism, electrolytes, and acid–base balance.[3]

3. If you suspect that opiates were also ingested, naloxone (Narcan) (0.4 mg, intramuscular [IM] or intravenous [IV]) should be given. If, as outlined in Section 6.2.3.2., the patient does not respond to two doses given within one-half hour, it is almost certain that opiates were not part of the respiratory and cardiac depression.

4.2.4. Psychosis (See Sections 1.6.4., 2.2.4., and 5.2.4.)

4.2.4.1. The Clinical Picture

The chronic ingestion of alcohol can cause suspiciousness that can progress to the point of frank paranoid delusions, that is, *alcoholic paranoia*. Similarly, alcohol can cause persistent hallucinations, usually voices accusing the patient of being a bad person or a homosexual (although at times the hallucinations can be visual or tactile), an example of *alcoholic hallucinosis.* Both pictures can develop in the midst of a drinking bout, occur in an otherwise clear sensorium (i.e., there's no organic brain syndrome), begin during alcoholic withdrawal, or have an onset within several weeks of the cessation of drinking. Both run a course of complete recovery within several days to several weeks if no further drinking occurs.[4] Clinically the syndrome resembles the stimulant-induced psychosis (see Section 5.2.4.) and psychoses associated with other depressant drugs (see Section 2.2.4.). It is not a form of schizophrenia, as there is no increased family history of that disorder in these individuals, and there is no evidence that alcoholic paranoia or hallucinosis progresses to schizophrenia.[5]

4.2.4.2. Treatment

1. If the patient has no insight into his delusions or hallucinations (i.e., he believes that they are real), he should be hospitalized to protect him from acting out his delusions.

2. Treatment should be aimed at giving the patient insight and at evaluating and treating any medical problems associated with his heavy intake of alcohol.

3. While the picture will clear spontaneously within a few days or several weeks, an antipsychotic agent like haloperidol (Haldol) at 1–5 mg per day (but up to 20 mg each day, if needed) by mouth may help keep the patient comfortable until the psychosis clears. There is no indication for continued use of these drugs, and they should be stopped within two weeks. If the patient has demonstrated delusions and/or hallucinations prior to the onset of heavy drinking or has a history of the psychosis persisting despite abstinence, the diagnosis of primary schizophrenia with secondary alcohol problems should be entertained and antipsychotic medications continued.[6]

4.2.5. Organic Brain Syndrome (See Sections 1.6.5., and 2.2.5.)

4.2.5.1. The Clinical Picture

Alcohol can cause mental confusion and clouding of consciousness through the direct effects of the drug, alcohol-related vitamin deficiencies, and indirect consequences of alcohol intake, such as trauma and metabolic disturbances.

4.2.5.1.1. Alcohol's Direct Effects

1. *Acute.* At relatively low doses, judgment and performance are impaired, but at blood-alcohol levels in excess of 150 mg %, a picture of confusion and disorientation occurs for most nontolerant people. The

OBS can be seen at even lower doses for the elderly and for individuals with preexisting brain disorders. The course is relatively benign, with a clearing of confusion occurring as blood-alcohol levels decrease.

2. *Chronic* heavy doses of alcohol are associated with a number of organic pictures, some of which may be permanent. As noted previously, 15–30% of nursing-home patients with chronic OBS have histories of alcoholism. This may result in part from the deleterious effects of alcohol on nerve cells, but it is also probably the combined result of alcohol, vitamin deficiencies, and trauma. The clinical picture and treatment would be similar to that of vitamin-related organicities as discussed below.

4.2.5.1.2. Vitamin Deficiencies

In the presence of alcohol, the body does not absorb thiamine adequately and uses what thiamine there is at a faster rate. This may be of great importance, especially to individuals with inefficient thiamine-dependent enzymes.[7] The result is a syndrome consisting of a mixture of neurological problems, such as ataxia, nystagmus, paralysis of certain ocular muscles, etc., characterizing Wernicke's Syndrome and psychological symptoms like markedly decreased recent memory, confusion, a tendency to make up stories to fill in memory deficits (confabulation) known as Korsakoff's Syndrome. The Wernicke–Korsakoff Syndrome (or variations thereof) runs an unpredictable course, with a tendency toward rapid and complete improvement of most neurological signs with the administration of adequate thiamine, but with a slower resolution of the mental clouding and a possibly permanent OBS.[8]

4.2.5.1.3. Other Causes of Organicity in Alcoholics

Any individual presenting with confusion, disorientation, and decreased intellectual functioning should receive a thorough evaluation for trauma (and resultant subdural hematomas), infections, and metabolic abnormalities (especially glucose, magnesium, and postassium problems).

4.2.5.2. Treatment

1. The cornerstone of treatment rests with finding and treating the physical causes (e.g., infection, electrolyte abnormalities, consequences of trauma, etc.).

2. All patients should receive thiamine in doses of 100 mg IM daily for at least three days, followed by oral multiple-vitamin preparations.

3. Patients should be given good general nutrition and lots of opportunity to rest.

4. While improvement in the level of organic impairment is to be expected, the mental confusion may clear slowly, and it may not be possible to establish the exact degree of permanent intellectual deterioration for several months.

4.2.6. Alcoholic Withdrawal (See Section 1.6.6., 2.2.6., and 6.2.6.)

4.2.6.1. The Clinical Picture

This is an example of the *depressant withdrawal syndrome* and is almost identical to the discussion given under CNS depressants in Section 2.2.6. Figure 4.1 outlines a simple approach to the symptomatology expected during withdrawal.

4.2.6.1.1. History

Some withdrawal symptomatology can be expected in any alcoholic who has been drinking daily—even if he did not become intoxicated every day. The intensity of the symptoms is difficult to predict with any degree of certainty, but the approach described in Section 4.2.6.3.2., may be helpful.

The alcoholic may present with a clear history of alcohol abuse, but more often he comes to the physician with a variety of psychological or physical complaints, as described in Section 4.1.1. It is wise to have a high index of suspicion for possible alcoholic withdrawal in all new patients, but this is especially true for those presenting with any of the more obvious stigmata of alcoholism, ranging from a high red blood cell MCV (see Table 1.5) to those demonstrating liver failure, cancer of the esophagus, or cancer of the head and neck. When a patient presents with

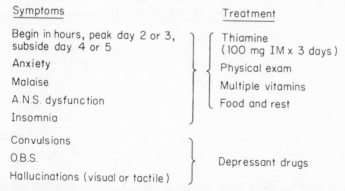

Figure 4.1. Detoxification. From Schuckit, M. A. Inpatient and residential treatments of alcoholism. In J. H. Mendelson & N. K. Mello (Eds.), *Diagnosis and Treatment of Alcoholism.* New York: McGraw-Hill, copyright © 1979. Reprinted with permission of McGraw-Hill Book Company.

any of the physical problems often associated with alcoholism or demonstrates a tremor and gives a history of alcohol misuse, the possibility of withdrawal must be carefully considered.

4.2.6.1.2. Physical Signs and Symptoms

The final clinical picture is a combination of any of the problems listed in Figure 4.1. Almost all individuals show some degree of anxiety, a drive to drink, tremor, and autonomic nervous system dysfunction (e.g., a pulse of 100–120, a temperature of 99°–100°F orally, respirations of about 25, and an unstable blood pressure). Only between 5% and 15% of the alcoholics going through withdrawal develop the more serious sequelae, including convulsions (these are drug-induced seizures not related to idiopathic epilepsy and not requiring chronic treatment) and OBS or hallucinations (usually visual or tactile and rarely auditory).[9-11]

4.2.6.1.3. Psychological State

This is as dramatic as the physical problems and consists of nervousness, a feeling of decrease of self-worth and a high drive to continue drinking and, for the 5–15% mentioned above, can include an obvious OBS or hallucinations.

4.2.6.1.4. Relevant Laboratory Tests

There are no laboratory tests that are pathognomonic for alcoholism. For an individual entering withdrawal, however, it is necessary to rule out all serious physical problems. Thus, it is important to perform an adequate neurological examination, to determine the cardiac status through an EKG, and to do any of the relevant laboratory procedures outlined in Table 1.5. Abnormalities in liver function and kidney function, as well as glucose levels, should be monitored throughout withdrawal but can be expected to return to normal within a week for most individuals unless serious permanent damage in the relevant organs has occurred.

4.2.6.2. Treatment

Therapy is rather simple and can be divided into identification of problems, offering general support, and carrying out active detoxification.

1. One of the most important steps is an adequate *medical examination* to rule out preexisting medical disorders that might complicate withdrawal and threaten life. There is a high risk of mortality if an individual

with serious physical damage enters a rather strenuous withdrawal without adequate treatment.[11] It is important to note the possibility of cardiac disorders, intracranial trauma, infections, and electrolyte abnormalities requiring specific treatment.

2. All individuals should be offered good general support, including adequate rest, good nutrition, and a generally supportive milieu.

3. The usual alcoholic going through withdrawal (except for those who evidence bleeding, persistent vomiting, or diarrhea) is *over*hydrated, not dehydrated.[12] Therefore, with rare exceptions, intravenous fluids *should not* be used and *ad lib* oral fluids should be relied upon to maintain adequate hydration.

4. It is especially important that all alcoholics receive thiamine in doses of 100 mg IM for one to three days, followed by routine daily oral multiple vitamins.[11]

5. It is possible at this point to begin education about the alcoholic process and attempt to convince the alcoholic to begin rehabilitation.

6. None of these generally supportive measures addresses the actual withdrawal syndrome. As is true with any physical addiction, one must recognize that physiological symptoms have occurred because the individual stopped the drug too abruptly. Therefore, one can administer the drug of addiction, or a cross-tolerant drug, in doses high enough to abolish symptoms and then decrease the drug slowly (in the case of alcohol, that can be a decrease of approximately 20% of the first day's dose each day).[11] This is especially important in dealing with the 5–15% of alcoholics who demonstrate convulsions, OBS, or hallucinations.

While any depressant drug, including alcohol, can be used,[13] I choose the benzodiazepines because of their relatively low rate of respiratory and blood pressure depression. Using chlordiazepoxide (Librium) as an example:

    a. I generally establish a prescribed oral dose of 25 mg three to four times a day initially.

    b. If the patient demonstrates obvious signs of withdrawal, such as a tremor, within an hour after administration of the drug, and if his blood pressure is relatively stable and he is awake and alert, an "as needed" (PRN) dose of 50 mg orally is given (the drug is poorly absorbed intramuscularly).[14]

    c. Each patient is titrated with PRN doses given for signs of withdrawal, but all doses are withheld if the patient develops a drop in blood pressure or excessive sleepiness. The total dosage on the first day is usually between 100 and 300 mg of chlordiazepoxide. Rarely, patients need even higher doses.

    d. The drug needed to diminish symptoms on the first day is then decreased by 20% each following day so that a patient requiring 200 mg on Day 1 would receive 160 mg on Day 2, 120 mg on Day 3, 80 mg on Day 4, etc.

    e. One advantage to chlordiazepoxide or diazepam (Valium) is the relatively long half-life, which (while necessitating special care to observe blood pressure depression and sleepiness in order to avoid overmedicating the patient) allows for a slow, steady decrease in blood drug levels and a resulting smooth withdrawal.

4.2.6.3. Some Withdrawal Treatment Variants[15]

4.2.6.3.1. The Social Model

The use of depressant drugs in treating the alcohol withdrawal syndrome requires that a physician and a registered nurse be available. In an effort to avoid the expense of such procedures, some programs choose to screen out patients with medical problems or those who appear to be heading for serious withdrawal and refer them to a hospital setting. This leaves the program with individuals who are likely to do relatively well (although showing signs of minor withdrawal) and who will respond to good general supportive care and milieu. In this model, although there is the possibility of serious medical complications, many more patients are reached at a lower cost than in a hospital setting.

4.2.6.3.2. Outpatient Detoxification

This approach to alcohol withdrawal also aims at saving money by the use of an *outpatient* alcohol withdrawal program. If one chooses to carry out detoxification outside of a hospital, it is imperative that *all patients be screened* for serious medical problems.[16,17] Next, a prediction of the final degree of withdrawal symptomatology is achieved by correlating present symptoms with the blood-alcohol level. Thus, an individual showing severe shakes and autonomic dysfunctioning with a rapidly decreasing blood-alcohol level of approximately 100 mg % can be expected to enter serious withdrawal and should be hospitalized, while another patient showing only minor tremors with a 0 blood-alcohol level is probably a good candidate for outpatient withdrawal.

During withdrawal, the patient is treated in a day-hospital setting and receives medication both at the hospital and from a friend or relative at home with medical backup by phone, if needed. A paradigm using chlordiazepoxide and a generally supportive milieu can be established similarly to that outlined above for inpatient detoxification.

4.2.7. Medical Problems

The deleterious effects of alcohol on alcoholics are so ubiquitous that it is impossible to discuss adequately all the resulting medical conditions in this short handbook. One is faced with recognition of the complications described in Section 3.2.2., and discussed in greater depth in a number of referenced texts.[18,19]

It is also important to consider alcohol-induced complications in nonalcoholics with chronic disorders. Examples include the increased chance of bleeding in individuals with ulcer disease, respiratory depression in people with emphysema, the adverse effects of alcohol on the livers of people with infectious hepatitis, the inference with normal pancreatic functioning for those who already have pancreatitis,[1] the deterioration in sugar metabolism that might adversely effect diabetics, and the impairment of cardiac functioning in individuals with heart disease.[20,21]

Alcohol also adversely effects the metabolism and efficacy of a wide variety of medications, including potentiation of the adverse effects of analgesics, adverse interactions with antidepressants, and interference with proper actions of all psychotropic medications.[20] The problems extend to antihypertensive drugs, as alcohol may potentiate orthostatic drops in blood pressure, and to hypoglycemic agents[21] and anticoagulants because of the induction of liver metabolic enzymes.

4.2.8. Other Problems

4.2.8.1. Pathological Intoxication

4.2.8.1.1. The Clinical Picture

This syndrome (which is probably both overdiagnosed and understudied) consists of the development of violent behavior at low doses of alcohol, usually followed by exhaustion and amnesia for the episode.[22,23] While this diagnosis is frequently included as part of a legal defense for individuals committing violent acts under the influence of ethanol, it is a relatively rare phenomenon and is seen primarily in individuals with evidence of organic brain damage.

4.2.8.1.2. Treatment

While no specific treatment regimen has been worked out, there are a number of common-sense suggestions.

1. The patient should be evaluated for a CNS epileptic focus, especially temporal lobe epilepsy.

2. Treatment in the midst of an episode is symptomatic and involves firm attempts to control behavior, using antipsychotics (such as haloperidol [e.g., 5 mg IM]) which may be repeated in one hour, if necessary.

3. All patients with this picture should be warned to abstain from drinking or, minimally, to avoid alcohol when they are tired, hungry, or under stress. They should be told that they are legally responsible for violent acts committed after voluntarily imbibing ethanol.

4.2.8.2. The Fetal Alcohol Syndrome

4.2.8.2.1. The Clinical Picture

Alcohol interferes with normal metabolic processes and the functioning of most organic systems and readily crosses the placenta to the developing fetus. Therefore, it is not surprising that there may be a direct correlation between the amount a pregnant woman drinks and the chance of her child's demonstrating problems, including a low birth weight, slow development, mental retardation, abnormalities in facial structure, cardiac ventricular septal defects, malformations of the limbs, etc.[24] In its full-blown form, the fetal alcohol syndrome may be seen in up to one-third of the children of *actively* drinking alcoholic women.

4.2.8.2.2. Treatment

The only treatment is prevention, and women should be advised not to drink at any time during pregnancy or, if they must drink, to keep the alcohol intake as low as possible.

REFERENCES

1. Schuckit, M. A. Alcohol and alcoholism: An introduction for the health care specialist. *Emergency Product News. 8*(5):26–30, 1976.
2. Perper, J. A. Sudden, unexpected death in alcoholics. *Alcohol Health and Research World.* Fall 1976:18–24.
3. Lowenstein, L. M., Simone, R., Boulter, P., *et al.* Effect of fructose on alcohol concentrations in the blood in man. *Journal of the American Medical Association. 213*(11):1899–1902.
4. Victor, M., & Hope, J. M. The phenomenon of auditory hallucinations in chronic alcoholism. A critical evaluation of the status of alcoholic hallucinosis. *Archives of General Psychiatry. 126:*451–481, 1955.
5. Schuckit, M. A., & Winokur, G. Alcoholic hallucinosis and schizophrenia: A negative study. *The British Journal of Psychiatry. 119*(552): 549–550, 1971.
6. Alpert, M., & Silvers, K. N. Perceptual characteristics distinguishing auditory hallucinations in schizophrenia and acute alcoholic psychosis. *American Journal of Psychiatry. 127*(3):298–302, 1970.
7. Blass, J. P., & Gibson, G. E. Abnormality of a thiamine-requiring enzyme in patients with Wernicke–Korsakoff syndrome. *New England Journal of Medicine. 297:*1367–1370, 1977.

8. Victor, M., Adams, R. D., & Collins, G. H. *The Wernicke–Korsakoff Syndrome.* Philadelphia: Davis, 1971.

9. Sellers, E. M., & Kalant, H. Alcohol intoxication and withdrawal. *New England Journal of Medicine.* 294(14):757–762, 1976.

10. Gessner, P. K. Failure of diphenlhydantoin to prevent alcohol withdrawal convulsions in mice. *European Journal of Pharmacology.* 27:120–129, 1974.

11. Smith, J. W. Medical management of acute alcoholic intoxication. *G.P.* 38(6):89–93, 1968.

12. Knott, D. H., & Beard, J. D. A diuretic approach to acute withdrawal from alcohol. *Southern Medical Journal.* 62:485–488, 1969.

13. Schmitz, R. E. The prevention and management of the acute withdrawal syndrome by the use of alcohol. Presented at the Annual National Council on Alcoholism meeting in San Diego, Calif., Apr. 29, 1977.

14. Greenblatt, D. J., Intramuscular injection of drugs. *The New England Journal of Medicine.* 295:542–546, 1976.

15. Peterson, B., *et al.* A medical evaluation of the safety of non-hospital detoxification. Prepared for National Institute on Alcohol Abuse and Alcoholism. National Technical Information Service, U.S. Dept. of Commerce. Springfield, Va., 1975.

16. Feldman, D. J., Pattison, E. M., Sobell, L. C., *et al.* Outpatient alcohol detoxification: Initial findings on 564 patients. *American Journal of Psychiatry.* 132(4):407–412, 1975.

17. Tennant, F. S., Jr. Ambulatory alcohol detoxification. *Newsletter from the California Society for the Treatment of Alcoholism and Other Drug Dependencies.* 4(1,2), 1977.

18. Becker, C. E., Roe, R. L., & Scott, R. A. *Alcohol as a Drug: A Curriculum on Pharmacology, Neurology and Toxicology.* Baltimore: Williams & Wilkins, 1974.

19. Morgan, R., & Cagan, E. J. Acute alcohol intoxication, the disulfiram reaction, and methyl alcohol intoxication. In B. Kissin & H. Begleiter (Eds.), *The Biology of Alcoholism. Volume 3: Clinical Pathology.* New York: Plenum Press, 1974, Chapter 5, p. 163.

20. Parker, B. M. The effects of ethyl alcohol on the heart. *Journal of the American Medical Association.* 228(6):741–742, 1974.

21. Pader, E. Clinical heart disease and electrocardiographic abnormalities in alcoholics. *Quarterly Journal of Studies on Alcohol.* 34:774–785, 1973.

22. Bach-Y-Rita, G., Lion, J. R., & Ervin, F. R. Pathological intoxication: Clinical and electroencephalographic studies. *American Jorunal of Psychiatry.* 127(5):698–703, 1970.

23. Maletzky, B. M. The diagnosis of pathological intoxication. *Journal of Studies on Alcohol.* 37(9):1215–1228, 1976.

24. Streissguth, A. P. Maternal drinking and the outcome of pregnancy: Implications for child mental health. *American Journal of Orthopsychiatry.* 47(3):422–431, 1977.

CHAPTER 5

Stimulants

5.1. INTRODUCTION

Stimulants are widely prescribed and greatly misused medications that have very limited bona fide medical uses. It is important that the clinician know these drugs well, as their misuse can mimic a variety of medical and psychiatric syndromes.

Abuse of stimulants has occurred for many centuries, beginning even before cocoa leaves were taken by natives of the Andes in South America.[1] Amphetamine itself was synthesized in 1887, with clinical properties recognized in about 1930, but until the middle 1950s or early 1960s this drug, as well as most stimulants, was felt to be generally safe. These claims were made despite evidence of the widespread misuse of cocaine in Germany after World War I[2] and epidemics of misuse of stimulants in Japan after World War II.[3]

5.1.1. Pharmacology (See Section 10.7., for over-the-counter stimulants.)

5.1.1.1. General Characteristics

The stimulants consist of a variety of drugs, some of which are outlined in Table 5.1, which share the ability to stimulate the CNS at multiple levels.[4] I will limit this discussion to those substances that are most clinically important, avoiding other stimulants (such as strychnine), which are not usually abused. As a group, the stimulants work, at least in part, by causing the release of neurotransmitters, (chemicals which stimulate neighboring neurons) such as norepinephrine from nerve cells. Some, in addition, can mimic the functions of transmitters like norepinephrine and have a direct effect upon nerve cells themselves. These include the analeptics, ranging from amphetamine through methylphenidate (Ritalin) to caffeine, and from cocaine (a local anesthet-

Table 5.1
Some Commonly Abused Stimulants

Generic	Trade
Amphetamine	Benzedrine
Benzphetamine	Didrex
Caffeine	
Chlorphentermine	Pre-Sate
Cocaine	
Dextroamphetamine	Dexedrine
Diethylpropion	Tenuate, Tepanil
Fenfluramine	Pondimin
Methamphetamine	Desoxyn, Fetamin
Methylphenidate	Ritalin
Phenmetrazine	Preludin
Phentermine	Ionamin, Wilpo

ic) to a variety of drugs touted for weight loss (e.g., phenmetrazine [Preludin]).

5.1.1.2. Predominant Effects

The most obvious actions of these drugs are on the CNS, peripheral nervous systems (outside the CNS), and cardiovascular systems. Clinically, the drugs cause euphoria, decrease fatigue and the need for sleep, may increase feelings of sexuality, interfere with normal sleep patterns, decrease appetite, increase energy, and tend to decrease the level of activity and distractibility in children with a hyperkinetic syndrome.[4]

Physically, the drugs produce a tremor of the hands, restlessness, and a rapid heart rate. Most of the substances have actions similar to amphetamine, although methamphetamine (Desoxyn) has less cardiac effects (especially at low doses), while methylphenidate (Ritalin) and phenmetrazine (Preludin) have lower levels of potency.[4,5] Cocaine, a local anesthetic and vascular constrictor, is quite potent, with effects similar to intravenous (IV) amphetamine.[6-8]

5.1.1.3. Tolerance and Dependence

5.1.1.3.1. Tolerance

Tolerance to stimulant drugs develops within hours to days as the result of both *metabolic* (a disturbance in drug distribution perhaps related to increased acidity of the body, acidosis) and *pharmacodynamic* tolerance (as exemplified by toleration of injections of up to 1 g of methamphetamine IV every two hours).[8] On the other hand, an important phenomenon of *reverse tolerance* can also be noted where *some* individuals show increasing effect of repeated doses of the medications, perhaps related to a CNS process similar to enhanced cellular sensitivity or kindling.[9] While there is a cross-tolerance between most of the stimulant drugs, it is not known whether this generalizes to cocaine.[8]

5.1.1.3.2. Physical Dependence

We are used to thinking of withdrawal symptoms as they relate to depressant and opiate drugs, expecting individuals to show anxiety, anorexia, or loss of appetite, sleeplessness, etc. Because of this, there has been a debate about whether actual physical withdrawal can be expected with stimulants; however, most investigators and clinicians feel that such a syndrome exists. This is described in detail in Section 5.2.6.

5.1.1.4. Purported Medical Uses

This section and Table 5.2 are included to reinforce the fact that despite the claim that stimulants are effective for many medical disorders, in most instances the potential benefit *does not* outweigh the potential harm. This is, at least in part, a consequence of the rapid development of tolerance which develops with stimulants, which seriously limits their ability to maintain a level of clinical usefulness.

Problems for which stimulants have been prescribed include:

5.1.1.4.1. Narcolepsy

This disorder, characterized by falling asleep without warning through the development of rapid eye movement (REM) or "dream-type" sleep at any time of the day or night, is associated with falling attacks (catalepsy). Stimulants can both modify and prevent attacks,[4] in

Table 5.2
Purported Medical Uses of Stimulants

Use	Comment
Depression	Stimulants can make the picture worse.
Dysmenorrhea	No proven usefulness.
Fatigue	Rule out medical diseases or depression. Stimulants do not work.
Hyperactive child syndrome	Very much overdiagnosed. Responds to stimulants or antidepressants.
Narcolepsy	A *rare* disorder that responds to other REM-suppressing drugs as well.
Obesity	Stimulants exert *temporary* relief. Dangers far outweigh assets

part by decreasing REM sleep. However, narcolepsy may be a very rare disorder and should be diagnosed only with brain wave or EEG studies, and other REM-decreasing drugs are available, including most of the antidepressants. Stimulants should be used very carefully, if at all, with this disorder.

5.1.1.4.2. The Hyperkinetic Child Syndrome (HS)

This syndrome of children and perhaps adults is characterized by a short attention span and an inability to sit quietly, with resultant difficulty in learning, and may be associated with signs of minimal brain damage.[10] However, hyperactivity is a common reaction to stress in childhood, and the diagnosis should not rest solely with the rapid evolution of a symptom of overactivity, especially when it occurs in relationship with a life problem.[11] This disorder, which appears prior to age 6, becomes much more incapacitating once school begins. For a bona fide HS, stimulants have been shown to be effective in decreasing symptomatology and increasing the ability to learn. In addition, carefully prescribed medication does not predispose the child to go on to drug abuse.[12] This is probably the only disorder for which stimulants are the primary drug of choice, but alternate modes of pharmacotherapy, including antidepressants, are available.[13]

5.1.1.4.3. Obesity

Stimulants do decrease the appetite, but only temporarily, with activity lasting *at most* three or four weeks.[14] In almost all controlled investigations, weight lost while on stimulants reappears within a relatively short period of time after the drug is stopped. Thus, considering the abuse potential of these drugs, their use in weight reduction is contraindicated.

5.1.1.4.4. Other Problems

The stimulants have also been used for *fatigue, depression, menstrual pain* or *dysmenorrhea,* and some *neurologic disorders.* Controlled studies have demonstrated that the drugs are not effective for these problems, and their potential dangers outweigh their usefulness.

5.1.2. Epidemiology and Patterns of Abuse

Enough stimulants are manufactured legally to give 50 doses each year to every man, woman, and child in the United States,[15] with an estimated one-half of this drug finding its way into illegal channels.[15] This availability, when added to the drugs that enter the country illegally (e.g., cocaine), and other drugs coming from illegal manufacturing sources, allows for high levels of stimulant abuse.

While extremely dangerous, the stimulating and euphoria-producing properties of the stimulants make them very appealing drugs. It has been estimated, for example, that the major limiting factor in the abuse of cocaine in the United States has been its high cost and limited availability. Nonetheless, at least 15% of all psychoactive drugs sold in the United States are amphetamines, and 15% of patients admitted to metropolitan psychiatric hospitals have traces of amphetamine in their urine.[3]

As with CNS depressants, abusers of these substances can be rather simplistically divided into those more middle-class individuals receiving the drug on prescription from one or a variety of physicians (medical abusers) and the predominantly young population primarily misusing drugs obtained from street suppliers or friends (street abusers). For either group, the drugs can be used alone or in an attempt to modify the effect of other substances, usually CNS depressants as described in Chapter 11. These drugs also appear to be used more and more in middle-class social settings as part of an attempt to increase a party "high."

5.1.2.1. Medical Abusers

These individuals usually begin using the medications for weight reduction, treatment of fatigue or dysmenorrhea, to study for exams, or to aid in long-distance drives. The patient may get all his drug from one physician, attempting to obtain multiple or refillable prescriptions, or he may receive simultaneous supplies from a variety of medical resources. In this setting, anecdotally, abuse tends to begin with a slow escalation of the dose, perhaps in response to the sadness, fatigue, and increased appetite that are seen when tolerance develops. Attempts at stopping the medication result in fatigue and an increased need for sleep, hypersomnia, leading, in turn, to drug dose escalation.

A related pattern of social abuse is seen in students, individuals working odd hours, truck drivers, and other people with abnormal sleep cycles or the need to get a large job done in a short period of time without much sleep. Under these settings, fatigue and depression secondary to stimulants are almost certain to develop, with some individuals also demonstrating paranoia, emotional lability, and even violence.

5.1.2.2. Street Abusers

Here, an individual is attempting to achieve an altered state of consciousness by taking oral, IV, or inhaled drugs. In one pattern, the person chronically misuses the drug either alone or in combination with depressant medications. In another mode, the person initiates repeated periods of "runs" of taking the drug around the clock for two to four days. Problems with withdrawal and psychosis can occur with any method of drug administration and pattern but are most likely to be seen with the IV method during a "run."

5.1.3. Establishing the Diagnosis

Any substance that so thoroughly mimics other medical and psychiatric emergencies and that is so readily available both on prescription and "on the street" must be considered part of the differential diagnosis in most emergency room situations. As with the other drugs of abuse, one must have a high index of suspicion or the diagnosis will be missed.[16] Because it is important to gather a careful history from both the patient and any available resource person about the use of stimulant drugs, I ask each patient about his pattern of prescription and illegal drug-taking.[16] I ask specifically about stimulants when an individual presents with any of the following problems[17]:

1. A restless, hyperalert state
2. An anxietylike attack (usually nervousness plus a rapid pulse)
3. A high level of emotional lability or irritability
4. Aggressive or violent outbursts
5. Paranoia or increased levels of suspiciousness[18]
6. Hallucinations, especially auditory or haptic (touch)
7. Confusion or an organic brain syndrome
8. Depression
9. Lethargy
10. Any evidence of IV drug use, such as needle marks or skin abscesses
11. Abnormalities in the nasal lining or mucosa such as might be expected with inhaling stimulants
12. Worn down teeth (from tooth grinding while intoxicated)

Also, in an emergency room, any individual presenting with *dilated pupils, increased heart rate, dry mouth, increased reflexes, elevated temperature, sweating,* or *behavioral abnormalities* should be considered a possible stimulant-drug misuser.[6,17] Under such circumstances, or if there is a hint of stimulants from either the patient or the family, it is a good idea to take blood or urine for a toxicologic screen.[19]

5.2. EMERGENCY PROBLEMS

The most frequently seen clinical problems associated with stimulant abusers are the panic reaction (frequently presenting as a pseudo-heart attack), a temporary psychosis, and medical problems.

5.2.1. Panic Reaction

5.2.1.1. Clinical Picture (See Sections 1.6.1., 7.2.1., 8.2.1., and 12.2.)

Stimulant drugs can give rise to at least two related forms of panic. In the first instance, the individual, even when taking stimulants in relatively "normal" doses, can experience a rapid heart rate, palpitations, anxiety, nervousness, and hyperventilation (the last resulting in altered blood carbon dioxide [CO_2] levels). The subsequent chest pains, in combination with anxiety and palpitations as well as shortness of breath, can give the individual the feeling that he is having a heart attack.[1]

The second rather classical picture relates to the psychological anxiety and nervousness that can be associated with stimulants. In such instances, the individual may "panic," feeling that he is losing control or going crazy.

5.2.1.2. Treatment

Treatment involves careful evaluation to rule out medical or psychiatric disorders, reassurance, and time.

1. The patient should be evaluated for bona fide medical illness, including the possibility of a heart attack, hyperthyroidism, etc.

2. A careful history should be taken to rule out preexisting psychiatric disorders, especially anxiety neurosis or affective disorder.[20]

3. Bloods (10 ml) should be drawn or a urine sample taken (50 cc) for toxicologic tests.

4. If the first two points are negative, the patient should be told that his reaction is a result of the drug and that the effects should wear off over the next two to four hours.

5. The patient should be reassured that he will recover totally.

6. Of course, if stimulant misuse is a regular occurrence for the patient, he should be referred for evaluation and counseling to an outpatient drug treatment program or an interested health professional.

7. Medications should be used sparingly, if at all. If needed, the antianxiety drugs (e.g., chlordiazepoxide [Librium], 10–25 mg by mouth, repeated several times in 30–60 minutes, if necessary) may be helpful.

5.2.2. Flashbacks

The relatively short length of action and the rapid metabolism of stimulants does not make them conducive to the development of flashbacks.

5.2.3. Toxic Reaction (See Sections 2.2.3,. 4.2.3., 6.2.3., and 12.4.)

5.2.3.1. The Clinical Picture

5.2.3.1.1. History

The patient is usually a member of the "street" culture, where abuse may be oral or IV, has a high-risk job (e.g., a truck driver or a student at exam time), or has a history of some "medical" use of stimulants. The clinical picture may develop within minutes (e.g., with IV use or "snorting") or more slowly over hours to days, as with oral use in cross-country truck drivers.

5.2.3.1.2. Physical Signs and Symptoms

Evidence of sympathetic nervous system overactivity dominates the clinical picture. Thus, the patient presents with a rapid pulse, an increased respiratory rate, and an elevated body temperature. At high levels of overdose, the picture progresses to *grand mal convulsions*, markedly elevated blood pressure, and a very high body temperature—all of which can lead to cardiovascular shock.[17] It has been estimated that between 100 mg and 200 mg of dextroamphetamine can be lethal in a nontolerant individual, but chronic users may tolerate 1 g or more.[6] Death, though infrequent, is usually related to a CNS vascular strokelike picture, cardiac arrhythmias, or high body temperature.[1-17] There may also be signs of IV drug use (e.g., needle marks or abscesses), or, if the patient takes the drug nasally, there may be an inflammation of the nasal mucous membranes or, with cocaine, a destruction of all or part of the nasal septum.

5.2.3.1.3. Psychological State

Taken in excessive doses, stimulants produce restlessness, dizziness, loquaciousness, irritability, and insomnia. These may be associated with headache, palpitations, and the physical signs and symptoms listed above. As the dose increases, toxic behavioral signs develop, including a high level of suspiciousness, repetitive stereotyped behaviors, grinding of the teeth (bruxism), repetitive touching and picking at various objects and parts of the body (stereotypy), and the repetitious dismantling of mechanical objects, such as clocks.[8]

5.2.3.1.4. Relevant Laboratory Tests

With the exception of a toxicologic screen and the usual vital sign changes expected with stimulants, there are rarely dramatic laboratory test results.

5.2.3.2. Treatment

The treatment chosen will depend upon the clinical condition of the patient at the time he comes for treatment.

1. Emergency care to ensure a patent *airway, circulatory* stability, and treatment of *shock* should be carried out as described in Sections 2.2.3.2., 6.2.3.2., and 12.4.

2. For an *oral overdose,* gastric lavage through either a nasogastric tube (for a conscious patient) or after intubation (for a comatose patient) should be carried out.

3. *Elevated body temperature* must be controlled, with all fevers above 102°F orally being treated with cold water, ice packs, or a hypothermic blanket.

4. *Repeated seizures* should be treated with IV diazepam (Valium) of from 5 to 20 mg injected *very slowly* intravenously over a minute and repeated in 15–20 minutes as needed. In this instance, intubation should be strongly considered, as IV diazepam could result in laryngospasm or apnea.[23]

5. A major elevation in *blood pressure* (e.g., a diastolic pressure of over 120 mm) lasting for over 15 minutes requires the usual medical regimen for malignant hypertension, which includes phentolamine (Regitine) IV drip of 2–5 mg given over 5–10 minutes as noted in Section 12.5.4.1 Failure to treat this symptom vigorously could result in CNS hemorrhage.

6. To help *excretion* of the stimulant, the urine should be acidified with ammonium chloride with the goal of obtaining a urinary pH below 6.6. This usually requires 500 mg orally every three to four hours.[16]

7. *Hyperthermia* and marked *agitation* can be treated with a dopamine-blocking agent such as haloperidol (Haldol) beginning with doses of 5 mg orally per day, but the dose might have to be a good deal higher for some individuals.[24] An alternate drug is chlorpromazine (Thorazine) in doses of 25–50 mg IM or orally to be repeated in 30–60 minutes, if needed, but in this instance one must be especially careful to avoid precipitating an anticholinergic crisis (see Section 10.2.4.2.) or a severe drop in blood pressure.[17] This, once again, underscores my preference for avoiding medications unless absolutely needed.

8. Patients rarely require dialysis, even though most of these drugs would respond to such measures if needed (see Section 12.4.3.2.).

9. Bloods and urines should be drawn for baseline studies and toxicologic tests. This will help you to rule out the concomitant use of other medications.

10. Once the patient begins to recover or if the overdose was not medically very serious, he should be placed in a quiet room with a minimal amount of stimulation.

11. Treatment of unintentional overdoses by children require basically the same approach.[25]

5.2.4. Psychosis (See Sections 1.6.4., 2.2.4., and 4.2.4.)

The stimulant-induced psychosis is a temporary but potentially dramatic picture.

5.2.4.1. The Clinical Picture

A high level of suspiciousness and paranoid delusions in a *clear sensorium* (the patient is alert and oriented) developing after an individual takes stimulants is called an *amphetamine* or *stimulant psychosis*.[15,16,19] This picture usually develops gradually with chronic abuse, although it can be seen acutely with one very large amphetamine dose.[17,18] The psychosis has been noted in normal volunteers when 10 mg of dextroamphetamine was given in slowly escalating doses.[26,27] The paranoia is usually associated with hallucinations, either auditory or haptic (the individual feels things crawling on him), but it can also be seen with visual hallucinations or illusions[16] and is usually accompanied by a very labile mood.[16,17,22] This picture often contains repetitive compulsive behavior.

The paranoid delusions can be very frightening to the patient. The level of insight or understanding is usually limited or nonexistent, and the suspiciousness has been known to result in unprovoked violence to the point of murder.[28] For instance, it has been reported that in the midst of the epidemic of amphetamine abuse in Japan, 30 of the 60 convicted cases in a two-month period were related to abuse of amphetamines.

With cessation of stimulants, the psychosis clears within two days to a week, the hallucinations disappearing first and the delusions later.[8,17,22] This is followed by increased sleep (usually accompanied by disturbing dreams) and a depression that may last two weeks or longer.[17]

The psychosis mimics an acute schizophrenic picture or mania. However, schizophrenia, as defined by Woodruff *et al.*,[20] has a relatively slow onset and is usually associated with a stable, somewhat bland mood; also, a schizophrenic rarely shows abnormal physical findings. On the other hand, a physical evaluation of the amphetamine psychotic can reveal severe weight loss, excoriations (from scratching at nonexistent bugs), needle marks, and elevated blood pressure, heart rate, and temperature.[16] These physical findings are quite variable, and their absence does not rule out amphetamine psychosis.

5.2.4.2. Treatment

Treatment of the amphetamine psychosis is relatively straightforward, as, even without active therapy, the pathological picture tends to disappear within days to a week.[8,17,22]

1. If the individual is out of contact with reality, it is best to hospitalize him.

2. The patient should be carefully screened for any signs of serious physical pathology, as a psychosis can be part of an overdose. A discussion of the treatment of the overdose is given above in Section 5.2.3.2.

3. Vital signs must be carefully recorded and blood pressures, especially those over 120 diastolic, should be treated with drugs such as phentolamine (Regitine) in doses of 2–5 mg given over 5–10 minutes. Special care must be given to avoid precipitating hypotension.[29]

4. In evaluating the clinical picture, consider the possibility that the individual may have also been abusing depressants and check for signs of depressant withdrawal.

5. In general, the patient should be placed in a quiet, nonthreatening atmosphere and should be treated with the general precautions one would extend to any paranoid patient (e.g., not performing any procedures without thorough explanation, not touching the patient without permission, and avoiding any rapid movements in the patient's presence).[16]

6. The treatment personnel should assume an appearance of self-confidence, but the possibility of unprovoked or assaultive behavior should be noted.[17]

7. As is true in a toxic reaction, it is possible that the administration of ammonium chloride (500 mg every three to four hours) to acidify the urine might help cut short the psychosis.[16]

8. A careful history of preexisting psychoses, especially schizophrenia or a serious manic or depressive disorder, should be taken from the patient and available resource people.

9. While my preference is to avoid medications, if behavior cannot otherwise be controlled, drugs can be considered.

     a. Some authors recommend chlorpromazine (Thorazine) in doses of 50–150 mg by mouth or 25–50 mg IM,[29] to be repeated up to 4 times a day, if needed, with special care to avoid anticholinergic problems or hypotension.[6,24] I avoid this drug as it tends to increase the half-life of amphetamine.[24]

b. Others recommend the use of haloperidol (Haldol) in doses beginning with 5 mg per day up to 20 mg daily given orally or IM.[24] As would be true with chlorpromazine, the drug need be given for only three to four days.

c. Some authors recommend the use of diazepam (Valium) in doses of 10–30 mg orally or 10–20 mg IM to control anxiety or overactivity.[29] However, I feel that there is no place for CNS-depressant drugs in treating the amphetamine psychosis, and they may increase the risk of violence.[24]

10. Patients should be referred after discharge to a drug treatment center to help them deal with their drug problems and to rule out the existence of other psychiatric disorders.

5.2.5. Organic Brain Syndrome

Confusion and disorientation can develop when an individual takes so much of the drug that his normal mental processes are disturbed.

5.2.5.1. The Clinical Picture (See Section 1.6.5.)

The organicity tends to be a transient problem consisting of any of the following symptoms including confusion, disorientation, hallucinations, delusions, paranoia, loose association of ideas, and behavioral problems of bruxism and repeated touching or stereotypic behavior.[8] It should be noted that the stimulants may cause cerebrovascular changes when taken chronically, and there are reports of increased rates of cerebral hemorrhage, subarachnoid bleeding, subdural hematomas, and vascular lesions resembling periarteritis nodosa in stimulant misusers.[30] There is also some *anecdotal* evidence that abusers of amphetamine and other stimulant drugs demonstrate a potentially permanent decrease in mentation and concentration.[15,30] Thus, abuse of stimulant drugs should be considered a part of the differential diagnosis of any individual presenting with signs of CNS organicity, and it is important that one carefully evaluate the neurological functioning of all stimulant misusers seen in practice.

5.2.5.2. Treatment

1. Because the organicity tends to be transient, the general approach is to give supportive care following the guidelines offered in Section 5.2.4.2.

2. However, one must be certain to carry out an adequate neurological examination to rule out all of the possible causes of an OBS, including a focal CNS lesion or intracranial bleeding.

3. One can roughly estimate the prognosis by determining which, if any, preexisting psychiatric disorder is present or if evidence of brain malfunctioning was present before the onset of the drug-induced problem.

5.2.6. Withdrawal

5.2.6.1. The Clinical Picture

5.2.6.1.1. History

Depending on the type of abuse involved (e.g., "street" versus medical), the patient may give an obvious history of drug abuse, or a great deal of probing and gathering information from friends and relatives may be required to establish the accurate diagnosis. The withdrawal may begin insidiously, with the patient's having no idea why he is depressed, lethargic, or irritable, or it may have a more dramatic onset.

5.2.6.1.2. Physical Signs and Symptoms

There is usually no specific physical pathology present, other than the usual type medical problems seen in any abuser. The withdrawal syndrome can begin while the individual continues to take stimulants as tolerance develops, and it may include a variety of nonspecific muscular aches and pains.[6,8]

5.2.6.1.3. Psychological State

Repeated administration of stimulants results in bad dreams as a result of the body's need to make up for the rapid eye movement (REM) sleep deprivation caused by stimulants. Feelings of sadness and hopelessness can be severe, sometimes leading to suicide, and the apathy and fatigue can last up to four weeks or more.[6,16] It is possible (but not definite) that some sadness and lethargy persist as a secondary abstinence syndrome over a period of months.

5.2.6.1.4. Relevant Laboratory Tests

There are no specific laboratory tests that will help here. Of course, all IV drug abusers should be screened for possible hepatitis (e.g., the liver function tests listed in Table 1.5) and signs of occult infection (a white blood count as listed in Table 1.5), and they should be given a good neurological examination (see Section 6.2.8.). A toxicologic screen may be helpful, but the signs of withdrawal might not appear until the stimulant drugs have been metabolized.

5.2.6.2. Treatment

Treatment is simply addressing the *symptoms,* as the major acute syndrome tends to dissipate in one to three days on its own (except for the depression and lethargy).

1. The patient must be given a careful neurological and physical examination.

2. The possibility of concomitant misuse of other drugs, especially depressants, must be considered. Bloods and urine samples should be sent for toxicologic screening and the patient carefully queried about other drug use.

3. A careful history of the drug misuse pattern and prior psychiatric disorders must be obtained.

4. The patient should be placed in a quiet atmosphere and allowed to sleep.[16]

5. If the patient is markedly despondent, (temporary) suicide precautions should be considered.

6. While, once again, I prefer to avoid medications, some authors suggest the use of haloperidol (Haldol) up to 5 mg a day (rarely up to 20 mg) for three days to a week to help modify symptoms.[16,17]

7. In general, allowing the person several days to recover and having him sleep and eat as much as he needs will usually result in the disappearance of all symptoms.

5.2.7. Medical Problems

The medical problems associated with overdose have been described in Section 5.2.3. Additional problems that must be considered are as follows:

1. Complications from the use of contaminated needles include endocarditis, tetanus, hepatitis, emboli, abscesses, etc. (see Section 6.2.8.).

2. Apparent signs of a stroke can accompany the strong contraction of blood vessels caused by stimulants.

3. A related phenomenon occurs in those individuals who sniff cocaine. The constriction of blood vessels in the nasal mucosa can be so severe that the nasal septum is destroyed.

4. The elevated blood pressure that can accompany the use of stimulant drugs can cause an intracranial hemorrhage.

5. The stereotyped behavior during intoxication can include grinding of teeth (bruxism), which can wear down the teeth and cause many dental difficulties.[1]

6. A variety of skin problems, including scratches (secondary to delusions about bugs in the skin) and skin ulcers, can be noted.

7. Individuals have been reported to develop temporary excessive movement of the lips, mouth, and face (dyskinesia).[1]

REFERENCES

1. Kramer, J. C. Introduction to amphetamine abuse. In E. H. Ellinwood & S. Cohen (Eds.), *Current Concepts on Amphetamine Abuse.* Rockville, Md.: National Institute on Mental Health, 1970, pp. 177–184.
2. Tatetsu, S. Methamphetamine psychosis. In E. H. Ellinwood & S. Cohen (Eds.), *Current Concepts on Amphetamine Abuse.* Rockville, Md.: National Institute on Mental Health, 1970, pp. 159–161.
3. Ellinwood, E. H., Jr. Amphetamine psychosis: Individuals, settings, and sequences. In E. H. Ellinwood & S. Cohen (Eds.), *Current Concepts on Amphetamine Abuse.* Rockville, Md.: National Institute on Mental Health, 1970, pp. 143–157.
4. Innes, I. R., & Nickerson, M. Norepinephrine, epinephrine, and the sympathomimetic amines. In L. S. Goodman & A. Gilman (Eds.), *The Pharmacological Basis of Therapeutics.* New York: Macmillan, 1975, pp. 495–503, 510–511.
5. Ayd, E. J. Protracted administration of methylphenidate (Ritalin). *Psychosomatics.* 5:180–187, 1964.
6. Medical Letter. Diagnosis and management of reactions to drug abuse. *The Medical Letter, Inc.* 19(3):13–16, 1977.
7. Ritchie, J. M., & Cohen, P. J. Cocaine: Procaine and other synthetic local anesthetics. In L. S. Goodman & A. Gilman (Eds.), *The Pharmacological Basis of Therapeutics.* New York: Macmillan, 1975, pp. 386–387.
8. Jaffe, J. H. Drug addiction and drug abuse. In L. S. Goodman & A. Gilman (Eds.), *The Pharmacological Basis of Therapeutics.* New York: Macmillan, 1975, pp. 302–305.
9. Post, R. M., & Kopanda, R. T. Cocaine, kindling and psychosis. *American Journal of Psychiatry.* 133(6):627–634, 1976.
10. Wender, P. H. Minimal brain dysfunction: An overview. In M. A. Lipton, A. DiMascio, & K. F. Killam (Eds.), *Psychopharmacology: A Generation of Progress.* New York: Raven Press, 1978, pp. 1429–1437.
11. Fish, B. The "one child, one drug" myth of stimulants in hyperkinesis. *Archives of General Psychiatry.* 25:193–203, 1971.
12. Schuckit, M., Petrich, J., & Chiles, J. Hyperactivity: Diagnostic confusion. *Journal of Nervous and Mental Disease,* 166:79–87, 1978.
13. Cohen, A. R. Tricyclic antidepressants and brain dysfunction. *Journal of the American Medical Association.* 225(2):177, 1973.
14. Maickel, R. P., & Zabik, J. E. The pharmacology of anorexigenesis. *Life Sciences.* 21:173–180, 1977.
15. Angrist, B. M., & Gershon, S. Psychiatric sequelae of amphetamine use. In R. I. Shader (Ed.), *Psychiatric Complications of Medical Drugs.* New York: Raven Press, 1972, pp. 175–199.
16. Tinklenberg, J. A. The treatment of acute amphetamine psychosis. In P. G. Bourne (Ed.), *A Treatment Manual for Acute Drug Abuse Emergencies.* Washington, D.C.: U.S. Government Printing Office, 1974, pp. 68–72.
17. Ellinwood, E. H., Jr. Emergency treatment of adverse reactions to CNS stimulants. In P. G. Bourne (Ed.), *A Treatment Manual for Acute Drug Abuse Emergencies.* Washington, D.C.: U.S. Government Printing Office, 1974, pp. 63–67.

18. Angrist, B. M., & Gershon, S. The phenomenology of experimentally-induced amphetamine psychosis—Preliminary observations. *Biological Psychiatry. 2:*95–107, 1970.
19. Connell, P. H. Clinical manifestations and treatment of amphetamine type of dependence. *Journal of the American Medical Association. 196*(8):130–135, 1966.
20. Woodruff, R. A., Goodwin, D. W., & Guze, S. B. *Psychiatric Diagnosis.* New York: Oxford University Press, 1974.
21. Suarez, C. A., Arango, A., & Lester, J. L., III. Cocaine-condom ingestion. Surgical treatment. *Journal of the American Medical Association. 238*(13):1391–1392, 1977.
22. Connell, P. H. *Amphetamine Psychosis. Maudsley Monographs #5.* London: Oxford University Press, 1958.
23. Model, D. G., & Berry, D. J. Effects of chlordiazepoxide in respiratory failure due to chronic bronchitis. *Lancet:*869–870, 1974.
24. Angrist, M.D., Less, H. K., & Gershon, S. The antagonism of amphetamine-induced symptomatology by a neuroleptic. *American Journal of Psychiatry. 131*(7):1974.
25. Espelin, D. E., & Done, A. K. Amphetamine poisoning. Effectiveness of chlorpromazine. *New England Journal of Medicine. 278*(25):1361–1365, 1968.
26. Griffith, J. D., Cavanaugh, J. H., & Oates, J. A. Psychosis induced by the administration of *d*-amphetamine to human volunteers. In D. H. Efron (Ed.), *Psychotomimetic Drugs.* New York: Raven Press, 1970, pp. 287–298.
27. Bell, D. S. The experimental reproduction of amphetamine psychosis. *Archives of General Psychiatry. 29:*35–40, 1973.
28. Ellinwood, E. H., Jr. Assault and homicide associated with amphetamine abuse. *American Journal of Psychiatry. 127*(9):1170–1176, 1971.
29. Dimijian, G. G. Differential diagnosis of emergency drug reactions. In P. G. Bourne (Ed.), *A Treatment Manual for Acute Drug Abuse Emergencies.* Washington, D.C.: U.S. Government Printing Office, 1974, pp. 1–8.
30. Grant, I., Mohns, L., Miller, M., & Reitan, R. M. A neuropsychological study of polydrug users. *Archives of General Psychiatry. 33:*973–978, 1976.

CHAPTER 6

Opiates and Other Analgesics

6.1. INTRODUCTION

This chapter is concerned with those pain-killing drugs (analgesics) that are most likely to be misused, ranging from propoxyphene (Darvon) through the synthetic, opiatelike drugs to the major opiates, including morphine and heroin. Historically, the widespread opiate abuse observed in Europe and the United States at the turn of the century was the result of legally purchased morphine and related compounds, primarily in middle-class women.[1,2] The preponderance of medical abusers of opiates continued until the drugs were placed under legal control in the early 1900s, after which the "street" misuse of these substances began, primarily in young men from poor areas. Since the mid-1960s, however, abuse of these substances has spread once again to the middle class, where the drugs are obtained through both physicians and the "black market."

6.1.1. Pharmacology (See Section 10.5., for over-the-counter analgesics.)

6.1.1.1. General Characteristics

The major opiates include natural substances, such as opium, morphine, and codeine; semisynthetic drugs produced by minor chemical alterations in the basic poppy products (e.g., heroin, hydromorphone [Dilaudid], and oxycodone [Percodan]); and synthetic analgesics, such as propoxyphene (Darvon), meperidine (Demerol), etc., as shown in Table 6.1. The relative potency of these drugs has been described in other texts and can be roughly gauged by the usual dosage, with a standard of 10 mg of morphine producing analgesia for the average individual.[3]

These drugs undergo similar metabolism in the body but differ in their degree of oral absorption (ranging from a low for heroin to a high for

Table 6.1
Opiate Analgesics

Drug type	Generic name	Trade name
Analgesics		
	Opium	
	Heroin	
	Morphine	
	Codeine	
	Hydromorphone	Diluadid
	Oxycodone	Percodan
	Methadone	Dolophine
	Propoxyphene	Daricin
	Meperidine	Demerol
	Diphenoxylate	Lomotil
	Pentazocine	Talwin
		Fortral
Antagonists		
	Naloxone	Narcan
	Nalorphine	Nalline
	Levallorphan	Lorfan
	Cyclazocine	
	Naltrexone	

propoxyphene). Heroin is rapidly converted by the body into morphine, with detoxification occurring primarily in the liver, and the resulting metabolites are excreted through the urine and bile. Over 90% of the excretion of doses of these drugs (with the exception of a very long-acting substance such as methadone) occurs within the first 24 hours, although metabolites can be seen for 48 hours or more.[3]

6.1.1.2. Predominant Effects

These substances all produce analgesia, drowsiness, changes in mood, and, at high doses, a clouding of mental functioning through depression of CNS and cardiac activity.[4] While there are some major differences in the way these drugs affect particular systems,[5] the actions are homogeneous enough to allow for some generalizations.

6.1.1.3. Tolerance and Dependence

6.1.1.3.1. Tolerance

Tolerance develops rapidly to most opiates, particularly the more potent analgesics, but the changes in organ sensitivity develop unevenly.[6] Almost all the opiates exhibit cross-tolerance to other members of the class.[6]

6.1.1.3.2. Dependence

These substances are very addicting, and physical dependence develops after relatively short-term use. The degree of dependence varies directly with the potency of the particular drug, the doses taken, and the length of exposure. Therapeutic doses of morphine given twice a day for two weeks or four times a day for three days can result in a mild withdrawal syndrome, especially if precipitated by a narcotic antagonist.[5]

6.1.1.4. Recent Findings on Brain Mechanisms

Recent discoveries on the pharmacology of opiates have been very exciting and are worthy of mention here. The work began with the hypothesis that there might be opiate receptors in specific areas of the brain. Logically, if there are endogenous opiate receptors, there must be endogenous opiates to occupy those receptors. This line of reasoning has resulted in the discovery of a series of substances (the endorphenes and enkephalens) that are present in various parts of the body, especially the CNS, and that appear to function in regulating the perception of pain. These substances have also been hypothesized to have some importance in the regulation of normal mood states, the development of psychoses, and the mediation of action of other misused substances. This series of investigations may lead to important breakthroughs in our understanding of the mechanism of action of these drugs, which might, in turn, lead to important information on the causes and treatment of substance misuse.[7,8]

6.1.2. Epidemiology and Pattern of Abuse

Simplistically, users divide into those who misuse analgesics in a medical setting *(medical abuse)* and those who take opiates obtained from nonmedical sources *(street abusers)*. The medical abusers tend to be older, middle-class, and well established in comparison to the street abusers, but there is much overlap between the two groups. Nonetheless, for clarity, the characteristics of street and medical abusers are (somewhat artificially) separated in this section.

6.1.2.1. Street Abuse

6.1.2.1.1. Pattern of Use

The sale of illicit opiates is a very profitable business. Most of these drugs enter the United States illegally as part of a highly complex economic/manufacturing ladder beginning in the Orient, the Middle East, or Mexico. The socioeconomics of heroin misuse have recently been outlined by Stimmel, demonstrating that 10 kg of opium grown from poppy plants at a cost of $250 results in street heroin worth $400,000 in the United States after a series of steps of manufacture and dilution with adulterants.[9] The resulting opiates are abused through all routes of administration, including oral (primarily the synthetic and semisynthetic opiates), intranasal (snorting), smoking (usually opium), and intravenous (especially heroin).[3]

The usual street abuser begins using opiates occasionally but progresses to daily use, with tolerance and physical dependence rapidly following. This pattern is certainly the one most likely to come to the attention of medical and mental health personnel as well as the police.

However, there are a number of individuals who continue to take the drug only occasionally over an extended period of time, even when used IV. The exact number of people "chipping" these drugs is not known, but it is probable that they show a much higher level of life stability with family, peers, and job than is true for the general user.[10]

A related phenomenon is seen in a number of physically addicted individuals who manage to hold jobs and function fairly well socially.[11] Another important observation grew out of Vietnam, where large numbers of soldiers with little or no prior experience with opiates found themselves in a situation of high stress with readily available drugs.[12] Under such circumstances, as many as one-half of those given the chance tried opiates, and while many became physically addicted, those who had not used drugs before Vietnam tended to return to a drug-free status when back in their home communities.[13]

6.1.2.1.2. The Natural History

The average street user tends to be young, a member of a minority group, and male.[14] He usually demonstrates a prior history of delinquent behavior (the more severe the antisocial problems, the greater the chance for continued drug use).[13] One recent study of a group of black addicts demonstrated that the average age of first use of any drug (usually marijuana) was 14, the first arrest for *any* problem occurred at 16.5, the first use of heroin at age 18, the first evidence of physical dependence at age 20, with the first heroin-related arrest following within about six months and the first treatment at approximately age 26.[14] Almost 80% of opiate addicts in treatment had early school problems, with 90% reporting truancy, two-thirds suspended from school, and 80% dropping out before graduating high school.[14] As was true in the discussion of alcoholism, individuals who qualify for the careful diagnosis of the antisocial personality (based on their antisocial behavior prior to age 16 and before the onset of serious drug misuse[15,16]) carry a much worse prognosis for violent behavior and continued drug and antisocial problems than the "average" street abuser.

The short-term prognosis for these individuals is relatively poor, with almost 90% returning to drugs within the first six months after treatment, but this return is followed by a trend toward an increasing percentage achieving abstinence over time.[17] Long-term follow-ups (up to 20 years) have demonstrated that a third or more of opiate abusers, even those severely enough impaired to be treated in a jail/hospital setting like the federal facility in Lexington, Kentucky, were finally able to achieve abstinence. The course for the remainder was far from benign, with one-quarter of the original total dead at follow-up and one-quarter still addicted.[18,19] The mortality rate for opiate abusers is about 5–10 per thousand, with especially high levels of death due to suicide, homicide, accidents, diseases, such as tuberculosis, and peripheral infections.[3] If remission is going to occur, it is probably seen after the age of 40,[20] but there is no absolute fixed age.[18] When an addict remains abstinent for three or more years, there is a very good chance that he will not go back to drugs.[18] Good prognostic signs for opiate addicts include a history of relatively stable employment, being married, a history of few delinquent acts, and few criminal activities unrealted to drugs.[13,17,18]

6.1.2.2. Medical Abuse

The medical-setting abusers have not been well studied, probably reflecting the fact that their use of opiates is not associated with a very high rate of unexpected death, serious crimes, or violence. What data there are indicate a preponderance of middle-class individuals, women, and those with pain syndromes.[21] The misuse is frequently one of multiple drugs, including depressants and stimulants as well as analgesics.

Two groups of individuals stand out at high risk for this syndrome. First, it has been suggested that a majority of those individuals with pain syndromes misuse their prescribed drugs.[21] The second important subgroup, health-care professionals (especially physicians and nurses), may have the highest rate of analgesic drug abuse of any middle-class population.[22] Possible explanations for this include the stresses of caring for other people's problems, the manner in which their job interferes with their ability to relate to their families, the long hours of their jobs, and the ready availability of drugs.

6.1.3. Establishing the Diagnosis

Diagnosis in either "street" or "medical" groups requires an awareness of the possibility of misuse with all patients[3] and a good medical history. In addition, there are a number of physical symptoms, signs, and behavioral patterns to watch for. These include:

1. *Increased pigmentation* over veins.
2. Evidence of clotted or *thrombosed veins.*
3. Other *skin lesions* and *abscesses.*
4. *Constricted* or small *pupils.*
5. *Swollen nasal mucosa* (if the drug was "snorted").
6. *Swollen lymph glands.*
7. An *enlarged liver.*
8. Abnormal laboratory tests, including *decreased globulins,* a positive *latex fixation test (VDRL), liver-function test* abnormalities, and a relatively high *white blood count.*
9. Evidence of visiting *multiple physicians* (perhaps to get a supply of drugs), a *complex medical history* that is hard to follow, or a de novo visit with complaints of *severe pain* (e.g., kidney pain, back pain, headache, abdominal pain, etc.), even with physical signs, as these are easy to produce at will (e.g., by placing a drop or two of blood in a urine sample).
10. Any *health professional* being seen for a syndrome for which analgesics might be prescribed.

6.2. EMERGENCY PROBLEMS

The most frequently occurring emergency difficulties seen with the opiates are toxic reactions and medical problems.

6.2.1. Panic Reactions (See Section 1.6.1.)

As is true of all the sedating drugs of misuse, individuals tend to be slowed down rather than panicked. Thus panic reactions rarely, if ever, occur.

6.2.2. Flashbacks

The relatively short half-life of most of these drugs and the rapid disappearance of the drug and the active metabolites make a flashback a rare phenomenon.

6.2.3. Toxic Reactions (See Sections 2.2.3., and 12.4.)

6.2.3.1. Clinical Picture

6.2.3.1.1. History

The opiate overdose is usually an acute, life-threatening event, with the patient found in a semicomatose condition with evidence of a recent IV injection (e.g., a needle in the arm or nearby) or empty bottles.

6.2.3.1.2. Physical Signs and Symptoms

The physical condition dominates the clinical picture. The specific symptomatology depends upon the drug, how long ago it was taken, and the patient's general condition. The range or symptomatology can include:

1. Decreased respirations.[23]
2. Blue lips and pale or blue body.
3. Pinpoint pupils (unless there is brain damage, in which case the pupils may be dilated).
4. Nasal mucosa hyperemia (for a patient snorting a drug).
5. Recent needle marks or perhaps a needle still in the arm.[23,24]
6. Pulmonary edema characterized by gasping, rattling respirations of unknown etiology (not related to heart failure), and a state of shock.[25]
7. Cardiac arrhythmias and/or convulsions, especially seen with codeine, propoxyphene (Darvon), or meperidine (Demerol).[24]
8. Death appears to occur from a combination of respiratory depression and pulmonary and/or cerebral edema.[3] The pulmonary edema may be related to an idiosyncratic reaction to the opiate or possibly an allergic response to either the drug or one of the adulterants (such as quinine) in the injected substances. There is no evidence that it is related to either a fluid overload or heart failure.[26] An alternate hypothesized mechanism is the possible development of cardiac arrhythmias, perhaps related to histamine release.

6.2.3.1.3. Psychological State

The patient is usually markedly lethargic or comatose.

6.2.3.1.4. Relevant Laboratory Tests (See Section 2.2.3.1.4.)

It is necessary to rule out all other causes of coma, such as head trauma (with a physical exam, a neurological exam, skull X rays, etc.), glucose or electrolyte abnormalities (as shown in Table 1.5), etc. The level of cardiac functioning must be established with an EKG and the level of brain impairment with an EEG, if appropriate. A toxicologic screen may be helpful.

6.2.3.2. Treatment (See Section 2.2.3.2.)

It has been suggested that the medical needs of the overdosed opiate abuser can be divided into emergency, acute, and subacute stages.[24,27] As outlined in Table 6.2, the general support first given addresses problems expected in any medical emergency. The levels of care listed here are not in a definite order and include:

1. Establish an adequate *airway; intubate* and place on a *respirator* if necessary using compressed air at a rate of 10–12 breaths per minute unless pulmonary edema is present.

2. Be sure the *heart* is beating; carry out external cardiac massage, defibrillate, or administer intracardiac adrenaline if needed; also, give 50 ml of sodium bicarbonate by IV drip for serious cardiac depression.

3. Prevent *aspiration* either by positioning the patient on his side or by using a tracheal tube with an inflatable cuff.

4. Begin an IV (large gauge needle) being prepared to replace all fluids lost to urine plus 20 ml per hour for insensible loss if the coma persists.

5. Deal with *blood loss* or hypotension with plasma expanders or pressor drugs as needed.

6. Treat *pulmonary edema* with positive-pressure oxygen, but beware of giving too much oxygen and thus decreasing the respiratory drive.

7. Treat *cardiac arrhythmias* with the appropriate drug.[28]

8. Administer a *narcotic antagonist:*

   a. *Naloxone* (Narcan) is the preferred drug, given in doses of 0.4 mg (1 ml) or .01 mg/kg IV and repeated in 3–10 minutes if no reaction occurs. Because this drug wears off in 2–3 hours, it is important to monitor the individual for at least 24 hours for heroin and 72 hours for methadone. Be prepared to deal with a narcotic abstinence syndrome, should you precipitate one with the narcotic antagonist (see Section 6.2.6.2.).

Table 6.2
Opiate Overdose: Symptoms and Treatment

Symptoms
    Unconscious and difficult to arouse
    Blue lips and body
    Small pupils
    Needle marks
    Pulmonary and/or cerebral edema
    Hypothermia
    Decreased respiration

Treatment
    Clear airway
    Artificial respiration
    Treat hypotension with expanders or pressors
    Treat arrhythmias
    Positive-pressure oxygen
    Naloxone 0.4 mg (1 ml) IV; repeat Q 2–3 h as needed
    Monitor 24+ hours

    b. If naloxone is not available, use *nalorphene* (Nalline), 3–5 mg IV (1 cc = 5 mg), repeated as necessary.

    c. If neither of these drugs is available, use *levallorphan* (Lorfan), giving 1 mg (1cc) IV,[27] repeating the dose in 10–20 minutes, if needed.

    9. Draw arterial *blood gases* if there are respiratory problems.

    10. Draw bloods for baseline *laboratory tests,* including CBC and the usual blood panel series as well as a toxicology screen (10 ml). If *hypoglycemia* is involved, administer 50 cc of 50% glucose IV.

    11. Establish *vital signs* every 5 minutes for 4 hours, with continued careful monitoring 24–72 hours.

    12. The more *subacute* and *chronic care* involves careful patient monitoring, dealing with *withdrawal signs,* treating *infections* (over one-half of individuals with pulmonary edema go on to develop pneumonia, but prophylactic antibiotics are not justified). You should continue to monitor vital signs and laboratory tests, and it is suggested that *tetanus* immunization be given.

    13. It is very important in treating the overdose to beware of the possibility of a *mixed drug ingestion.* These may require special measures, including the possible need for dialysis (see Section 12.4.3.2.).

6.2.4. Psychosis (See Section 1.6.4.)

Unlike most other drugs, the opiates are not known to produce any type of temporary psychosis.

6.2.5. Organic Brain Syndrome (See Section 1.6.5.)

This is unusual with opiates except as part of an obvious toxic overdose.

6.2.6. Opiate Withdrawal in the Adult (See Sections 2.2.6., and 4.2.6.)

The opiate withdrawal syndrome, seen for all of the analgesics discussed in this chapter including propoxyphene (Darvon), was one of the first well-described abstinence pictures (with the exception of alcohol). A somewhat arbitrary distinction between phases of withdrawal is outlined in Table 6.3. However, it is important to note that these phases overlap greatly.

Table 6.3
Acute Opiate Withdrawal (Heroin)[6]

Marked drive for the drug	Begins in hours, peaks in 36–72 hours.
Tearing Running nose Yawn Sweat	Begins 8–12 hours, peaks in 48–72 hours.
Restless sleep	Begins 12–14 hours, peaks in 48–72 hours.
Dilated pupils Anorexia Gooseflesh Irritability Tremor	Begins 12 hours, peaks in 48–72 hours.
Insomnia Violent yawn Weakness GI upset Chills Flushing Muscle spasm Ejaculation Abdominal pain	At peak.

6.2.6.1. The Clinical Picture

6.2.6.1.1. Acute Withdrawal

1. *History.* The onset of withdrawal usually begins at the time of the next scheduled drug dose, ranging from 4 to 6 hours for heroin to a day or more for methadone. The accurate diagnosis may be fairly obvious when the patient demonstrates the physical signs and symptoms as well as the psychological state described below and requests opiates, but frequently the clinician must have an index of suspicion and probe for potential "street" or medical abuse.

The most usual withdrawal syndrome of the "street" abuser is a relatively benign mixture of emotional, behavioral, and physical symptoms.[29] This is due to the variability in the potency of heroin obtained on the street, ranging from 0% to 77% (with most around 3%). Adulterants, such as lidocaine, procaine, quinine, lactose, etc., make up most of the substances sold as street opiates.[30]

2. *Physical signs and symptoms.* While a great degree of variability can be expected, it is possible to make the following generalizations:

    a. Within 12 hours of the last dose, there is usually the beginning of *physical discomfort*, characterized by tearing of the eyes, a runny nose, sweating, and yawning.

    b. Within 12–14 hours, and peaking on the second or third day, the patient moves into a *restless sleep* (a "yen").

    c. Over the same time period, other symptoms begin to appear including *dilated pupils, loss of appetite, gooseflesh* (hence, the term, *cold turkey), back pain,* and a *tremor.*

    d. This picture gives way to *insomnia;* incessant *yawning; a flulike* syndrome consisting of weakness, GI upset, chills, and flushing; *muscle spasm; ejaculation;* and *abdominal pain.*

    e. In the acute phases of withdrawal, the syndrome *decreases* in intensity and is usually greatly reduced by the fifth day, disappearing in one week to ten days.

    3. *Psychological state.* This is as important as the physical problems and includes a strong *"craving"* along with emotional *irritability.*

    4. *Relevant laboratory tests.* As the patient's degree of physical impairment tends to be less severe than that noted for the CNS depressants, it is usually enough to carry out a good physical exam and establish the baseline laboratory functions described in Table 1.5. A toxicologic screen may be helpful in establishing the recent use of opiates and analgesics.

6.2.6.1.2. Protracted Abstinence

The acute abstinence phase is followed by a more protracted abstinence, with two probable subphases.[3,6]

    1. The early phase of protracted abstinence lasts from approximately *Week 4 to Week 10* and consists of a mild increase in blood pressure, temperature, respirations, and pupillary diameter.

    2. This is followed by a later phase lasting 30 *weeks or more,* consisting of a mild decrease in all of the above measures and a decrease in the respiratory center response to carbon dioxide. It is possible to see differences in autonomic nervous system responses to opiates as long as one year after acute withdrawal is complete.[31]

Thus, what we recognize most clearly as withdrawal is only the acute phase. The protracted abstinence, consisting of physiological as well as behaviorally mediated aspects, goes on for many months. It is possible that this long-term syndrome produces a vague discomfort that may play an important role in driving the addict back to drug use.

6.2.6.2. Treatment (Review Section 2.2.6.2., as well.)

Treatment of the opiate withdrawal syndrome in adults is briefly outlined in Table 6.4 and in references 3, 6, 25, 30, and 32.

Table 6.4
Treatment of Opiate Withdrawal

General support
  Physical and laboratory exam.
  Rest.
  Nutrition.
  Reassurance.
  Honest appraisal of what is to be expected.
  Keep one doctor in charge.

One type of specific treatment
  E.g., methadone ≤ 15–20 mg orally as a test.
  Determine dose on day 1 or 2.
  Give dose BID.
  Decrease by 20%/day or over 2 weeks.

1. The first phase of therapy involves a good medical examination, as these patients have high rates of medical disorders as discussed below.

2. The physician must do all he can to develop a positive physician–patient contact to maximize patient comfort and cooperation. It is important that one physician be in charge.

3. After estimating the probable degree of dependence and thereby deciding whether active treatment of withdrawal is needed, it is important to explain carefully to the patient the symptoms he can expect and the fact that these cannot be totally eliminated. However, he should be reassured that you will do everything you can to minimize his discomfort.

4. You should establish a flow sheet of symptom severity and the treatments.[30]

5. The treatment of the physical withdrawal symptoms begins with the readministration of an opiate to the point where symptoms are greatly reduced, after which the drug dose is slowly decreased over a period of 5–14 days.

   a. Any opiate can be used, but most authors recommend oral methadone.

      i. Give a test dose of 20–50 mg of methadone orally and repeat the dose if symptoms are not alleviated, thus determining the minimum dose needed to control symptoms during the first 24–36 hours. Note that 1 mg of methadone roughly equals 2 mg of heroin or 20 mg of meperidine (Demerol).
      ii. Most addicts achieve some comfort at doses of 20 mg of methadone the first day. The necessary drug is then divided into twice-daily doses, with daily decreases of 10–20% of the

first day's dose, depending upon the development of symptomatology.

b. An alternate approach is to administer 10 mg of methadone IM and observe the effects, reexamining the patient in eight hours and monitoring the amount of drug necessary to abolish symptoms.[30] This makes it possible to determine the amount of drug needed to control symptoms in the first 24 hours, after which the doses can be given orally two to three times a day and decreased as described above.

c. It is possible to administer any opiate, establishing the necessary first-day dose and decreasing the drug by 10–20% per day. One example is propoxyphene (Darvon) treatment, where an initial detoxification dose of 800 mg per day has been used in a 21-day withdrawal program.[33]

d. A special case occurs when an individual has been taking part in a methadone maintenance program. Under these circumstances, it is advisable to decrease the drug slowly to minimize the chance of the development of symptoms. This usually means a diminution of approximately 3 mg from the daily dose each week, but even at this rate, some symptoms will be seen.

6. During detoxification, it is very important that some thought be given to plans for rehabilitation. It should be recognized that many patients enter detoxification solely to decrease their high drug levels or in response to immediate life problems. Under such circumstances, the individual may not want to participate in a rehabilitation program—only 10% of those who complete a detoxification program seek long-term care.[34] However, for those who might consider rehabilitation, the detoxification period is an excellent time to introduce them to the need for permanent abstinence, and counseling should be offered to *everyone*.

6.2.7. Opiate Withdrawal in the Neonate

A special case of opiate withdrawal is seen in the newborn, passively addicted by the mother's drug misuse during the latter part of pregnancy.[3,6] This addiction develops in the children of 50–90% of heroin-dependent mothers and carries a mortality of between 3% and 30%.

6.2.7.1. The Clinical Picture

The syndrome consists of *irritability, crying,* a *tremor* (seen in 80%), increased *reflexes,* increased *respiratory* rate, *diarrhea, hyperactivity* (seen in 60%), *vomiting* (seen in 40%), and *sneezing/yawning/hiccuping* (seen in

30%). The child usually has a *low birth weight* but may be otherwise unremarkable until the second day, when symptoms usually begin.

6.2.7.2. Treatment

1. A first step should be prevention. For those pregnant addicts on methadone maintenance, it is important that the drug be reduced to 20 mg a day or less during the last six weeks of pregnancy.[35]

2. Treatment of neonatal withdrawal consists of general support and observation, including keeping the child in a warm, quiet environment and observing electrolytes, glucose, etc.

3. In addition, the child with moderate to severe symptoms should be treated with any one of: *paregoric,* 2–4 drops per kg; *or methadone,* 0.1–0.5 mg per kg; *or phenobarbital,* 8 mg per kg; *or Valium,* 1–2 mg every 8 hours.[3,36,37] Medications should be given for 10–20 days, decreasing the amounts toward the end of that period.

4. It is also possible to treat, at least partially, the addicted infants of mothers on methadone maintenance by having them breast-feed while they continue to take their methadone. Additional drugs can be given to the child as needed.

6.2.8. Medical Problems

Opiate abusers, especially those taking street drugs, frequently present for care in some sort of medical crisis.[38] This may be an overdose or other serious medical problems as a consequence of the adulterants in opiate mixtures or the poor hygienic practices involved in the use of needles. A variety of texts have covered the medical problems and their treatment in detail.[3,30,38] These will be mentioned only briefly here. My goal is to increase your level of awareness of the problems so that you can then use the proper medical procedures.

Some of the more common problems include:

1. Abscesses and other infections of the skin and muscle
2. Tetanus or malaria
3. Hepatitis and other liver abnormalities
4. Gastric ulcers
5. Heart arrhythmias
6. Endocarditis
7. Anemias
8. Bone and joint infections
9. Eye-ground abnormalities, as they reflect emboli from the adulterant added to the street drug[39]
10. Kidney failure secondary to infections or adulterants

11. Muscle destruction
12. Pneumonia
13. Lung abscesses
14. Tuberculosis

In addition, addicts may present with a series of emotional and social problems, including:

15. Depression, frequently seen during methadone maintenance[40]
16. Sexual functioning abnormalities, which may partially reflect the transiently low testosterone level seen during chronic administration and lasting at least a month after the opiate is stopped[41]
17. Police problems
18. Social and interpersonal problems

These problems point out the absolute necessity for careful evaluation of medical and emotional problems in *any* opiate abuser undergoing treatment.

REFERENCES

1. Judson, H. F. *Heroin Addiction in Britain. What Americans Can Learn from the English Experience.* New York: Harcourt Brace Jovanovich, 1973.
2. Musto, D. F. *The American Disease. Origins of Narcotic Control.* New Haven, Conn.: Yale University Press, 1973.
3. Stimmel, B. *Heroin Dependency: Medical, Economic, and Social Aspects.* New York: Stratton Intercontinental Medical Book Corp., 1975.
4. Jaffe, J. H., & Martin, W. R. Narcotic analgesics and antagonists. In L. S. Goodman & A. Gilman (Eds.), *The Pharmacological Basis of Therapeutics.* New York: Macmillan, 1975, Chapter 15.
5. Lal, H. Minireview. Narcotic dependence, narcotic action and dopamine receptors. *Life Sciences. 17:*483–496.
6. Jaffe, J. H. Drug addiction and drug abuse. In L. S. Goodman & A. Gilman (Eds.), *The Pharmacological Basis of Therapeutics.* New York: Macmillan, 1975, pp. 286–324.
7. Snyder, S. H., Pert, C. B., & Pasternak, G. W. The opiate receptor. *Annals of Internal Medicine. 81*(4):534–540, 1974.
8. Bloom, F., Segal, D., Ling, N., *et al.* Endorphins: Profound behavioral effects in rats suggest new etiological factors in mental illness. *Science. 194:*630–632, 1976.
9. Stimmel, B. The socioeconomics of heroin dependency. *New England Journal of Medicine. 287:*1275–1280, 1972.
10. Zinberg, N. E., & Jacobson, R. C. The natural history of "chipping." *American Journal of Psychiatry. 133*(1):37–40, 1976.
11. Caplovitz, D. *The Working Addict.* New York: The Graduate School and the University Center of the City University of New York, 1976.
12. Dess, W. J., & Cole, F. C. The medically evacuated Viet-Nam narcotic abuser: A follow-up rehabilitative study. *Bulletin on Narcotics. 24*(2):55–65, 1977.

13. Robins, L. N., Helzer, J. E., & Davis, D. H. Narcotic use in Southeast Asia and Afterward. *Archives of General Psychiatry. 32:*955–961, 1975.
14. Halikas, J. A., Darvish, H. S., & Rimmer, J. D. The black addict: 1. Methodology, chronology of addiction, and overview of the population. *American Journal of Drug and Alcohol Abuse. 3*(4):529–543, 1976.
15. Woodruff, R. A., Goodwin, D. W., & Guze, S. B. *Psychiatric Diagnosis.* New York: Oxford University Press, 1974.
16. Robins, L. N. *Deviant Children Grown Up.* Baltimore: Williams & Wilkins, 1966.
17. Langenauer, B. J., & Bowden, C. L. A follow-up study of narcotic addicts in the NARA program. *American Journal of Psychiatry. 128*(1):73–78, 1971.
18. Vaillant, G. E. A 20-year follow-up of New York narcotic addicts. *Archives of General Psychiatry. 29:*237–241, 1973.
19. Snow, M. Maturing out of narcotic addiction in New York City. *The International Journal of the Addictions. 8*(6):921–938, 1973.
20. Winick, C. The life cycle of the narcotic addict and of addiction. *Bulletin on Narcotics. 26*(1):1–11, 1964.
21. Lass, H. Most chronic pain patients misuse drugs, study shows. *Hospital Tribune World Service.* 16, 1976, p. 2.
22. Jones, R. E. A study of 100 physician psychiatric inpatients. *American Journal of Psychiatry. 134*(10):1119–1122, 1977.
23. Kaufman, R. E., & Levy, S. B. Overdose treatment. Addict folklore and medical reality. *Journal of the American Medical Association. 227*(4):411–413, 1974.
24. Greene, M. H., & DuPont, R. L. The treatment of acute heroin toxicity. In P. G. Bourne (Ed.), *A Treatment Manual for Acute Drug Abuse Emergencies.* Washington, D.C.: U.S. Government Printing Office, 1974, pp. 11–16.
25. Medical Letter. *Diagnosis and Management of Reactions to Drug Abuse.* New Rochelle, N.Y.: The Medical Letter, Inc., Vol 19(3), Feb. 11, 1977.
26. Dimijian, G. G. Differential diagnosis of emergency drug reactions. In P. G. Bourne (Ed.), *A Treatment Manual for Acute Drug Abuse Emergencies.* Washington, D.C.: U.S. Government Printing Office, 1974, pp. 1–7.
27. Kleber, H. D. The treatment of acute heroin toxicity. In P. G. Bourne (Ed.), *A Treatment Manual for Acute Drug Abuse Emergencies.* Washington, D.C.: U.S. Government Printing Office, 1974, pp. 17–21.
28. Boedeker, E. C., & Dauber, J. H. (Eds.). *Manual of Medical Therapeutics,* 21st Ed. Boston: Little, Brown, 1974.
29. Siegel, S. Evidence from rats that morphine tolerance is a learned response. *Journal of Comparative Physiol. Psychology. 89:*498–506, 1975.
30. Shapira, J. *Drug Abuse: A Guide for the Clinician.* New York: American Elsevier, 1975.
31. Cohen, S. (Ed.). The drug schedules: An updating for professionals. *Drug Abuse and Alcoholism Newsletter. 5*(3), San Diego: Vista Hill Foundation, Apr. 1976.
32. Dole, V. P. Management of the opiate abstinence. In P. G. Bourne (Ed.), *A Treatment Manual for Acute Drug Abuse Emergencies.* Washington, D.C.: U.S. Government Printing Office, 1974, pp. 34–38.
33. Tennant, F. S., Russell, B. A., Casas, S. K., *et al.* Heroin detoxification. A comparison of propoxyphene and methadone. *Journal of the American Medical Association. 232*(10):1019–1022, 1975.
34. Sheffet, A., Quinones, M., Levenhar, M. A., *et al.* An evaluation of detoxification as an initial step in the treatment of heroin addiction. *American Journal of Psychiatry. 133*(3):337–340, 1976.
35. Strass, M. E., Andresko, M., Stryker, J. C., *et al.* Relationship of neonatal withdrawal to maternal methadone dose. *American Journal of Drug and Alcohol Abuse. 3*(2):339–345, 1976.

36. Ingall, D., & Zuckerstatter, M. Diagnosis and treatment of the passively addicted newborn. *Hospital Practice.* Aug. 1970, pp. 101–104.
37. Reddy, A. M. The management of the narcotic withdrawal syndrome in the neonate. In P. G. Bourne (Ed.), *A Treatment Manual for Acute Drug Abuse Emergencies.* Washington, D.C.: U.S. Government Printing Office, 1974, pp. 27–29.
38. Cherubin, C. E. Management of acute medical complications resulting from heroin addiction. In P.G. Bourne (Ed.), *A Treatment Manual for Acute Drug Abuse Emergencies.* Washington, D.C.: U.S. Government Printing Office, 1974, pp. 38–48.
39. AtLee, W. E. Talc and cornstarch emboli in eyes of drug abusers. *Journal of the American Medical Association. 219*(1):49–51, 1972.
40. Weissman, M. M., Slobetz, F., Prusoff, B., et al. Clinical depression among narcotic addicts maintained on methadone in the community. *American Journal of Psychiatry. 133*(12):1434–1438, 1976.
41. Mendelson, J. H., Mendelson, J. E., & Patch, V. D. Plasma testosterone levels in heroin addiction and during methadone maintenance. *The Journal of Pharmacology and Experimental Therapeutics. 192*(1):211–217, 1975.

Cannabinols

7.1. INTRODUCTION

Marijuana is second only to alcohol as the most widely used of the drugs described in this text. The health care problems involved with delta-9-tetrahydrocannabinol, or THC (the most active ingredient in marijuana and hashish) include panic reactions, toxic reactions, and a great deal of anxiety in the general population about possible mental and physiological damage to young users. Because, as health care deliverers, you will be called upon to give information about this drug to worried parents and to teenagers attempting to make decisions about future use, this chapter presents information on the history, physiology, and medical effects of the cannabinols.

THC is an ancient drug with use dating back to at least 2700 B.C.[1] It has been used in many cultures, including the Middle East, the Orient, and Western countries, where it has received a variety of names, ranging from hashish to charas, bhang, ganja, dogga, etc. In North America, THC is obtained as marijuana or hashish. (Pure THC is not available "on the streets," and samples so labeled are usually LSD or PCP—see Chapter 8.) At low to moderate doses, THC produces fewer physiological and psychological alterations than do most other classes of drugs, including alcohol. However, the fact that this drug does affect the nervous system, and that the peak age of use occurs in late adolescence when the brain is still developing, makes the substance a legitimate concern.

7.1.1. Pharmacology

THC comes from the marijuana plant, *Cannbis sativa*, which grows readily in warm climates—the percentage of active THC produced parallels the amount of sunlight received by the plant. Marijuana, the less potent source of THC, is the dried plant leaves, while hashish and other more potent sources of the drug are the resins of the plant flowers.

7.1.1.1. General Characteristics

While this drug is usually called a hallucinogen, at the doses most frequently taken the predominant effects are euphoria and a change in the level of consciousness without frank hallucinations. The drug can be ingested through smoking, eating, and (rarely) intravenous injection. The average cigarette contains 2.5–5.0 mg of the most active THC, delta-9-THC; however, only one-half of the drug is absorbed through this route of administration.[1] The potency of a cigarette depends upon the quality of the marijuana used (whether from the stems, leaves, or flowering tops, in increasing order of potency) and the amount of time elapsed since the plant was harvested (there is a decrease in potency over time[2]).

When it is smoked, the peak plasma level is reached within 10–30 minutes, with intoxication usually lasting between two and eight hours, depending upon the dose.[3] Eating the plant produces a greater percentage of the drug absorbed, with a resulting longer (but less predictable) "high." Here, the onset is seen in one-half to one hour, a peak blood level in two to three hours, with effects lasting up to eight hours.

There is no readily available manner of measuring THC levels in the blood. Once ingested, the drug tends to disappear from the plasma rapidly, becoming absorbed in tissues, especially those with high levels of fat, such as brain and testes.[1] The half-life is felt to be seven days,[4] primarily a result of THC in tissues, with active ingredients found for as long as eight or more days.[5] The drug is first metabolized to an 11-hydroxylated derivative with some psychoactivity; however, the remaining metabolites do not change levels of consciousness. THC is excreted primarily as metabolites, mostly in the feces, but also in the urine.[5] While the mechanism of action of THC is not well understood, there is some evidence for disruption of cellular metabolism and prevention of the proper formation of proteins, including DNA and RNA.[4]

7.1.1.2. Predominant Effects

The greatest effects of THC are on the brain, the heart or cardiovascular system, and the lungs. Most, if not all, changes occur acutely and appear to be reversible.

The changes in mood seen with THC depend not only on the amount of drug but also on the setting in which the substance is taken and, as with any more "mild" drug, what one expects to happen.[6] In addition to euphoria, the individual usually experiences a feeling of relaxation and sleepiness and heightened sexual arousal, is unable to keep accurate track of time, experiences hunger, and exhibits decreased social interaction. The user develops problems with short-term memory and may demonstrate an impairment in the ability to carry out multiple-step tasks.[1,7] Intoxication may be associated with mild levels of suspiciousness or paranoia along with some loss of insight.[8,9] If intoxication occurs during a state of high stress, a heightened level of aggressiveness might occur; however, most frequently one sees a decrease in this attribute.[7,8] At higher doses, frank hallucinations may occur, usually visual, sometimes accompanied by paranoid delusions. As with any toxic reaction, this can be associated with confusion, disorientation, and panic, as described in Section 7.2.

There are a variety of physiological problems that accompany moderate intoxication. These include fine shakes or tremors, a slight decrease in body temperature, a decrease in muscle strength and balance, a decreased level of motor coordination, dry mouth, and bloodshot eyes (injected conjunctivae).[1,7,10] Some individuals experience nausea, headache, nystagmus, and mild lowered blood pressure.[7,11] THC may also precipitate seizures in epileptics.[12]

Along with an increased breathing rate, the respiratory effects of acute administration of THC include increased diameters of bronchial tubes of potential significance in treating asthma.[7,12] However, chronic use results in a decreased rather than an increased diameter and a worsening of breathing problems.[4,13]

Marijuana affects the heart by increasing heart rate, resulting in an increased cardiac work load. Thus, this drug can be dangerous in individuals with preexisting cardiac disease.[14]

7.1.1.3. Tolerance and Dependence

7.1.1.3.1. Tolerance

Neither tolerance nor physical dependence is a major problem with marijuana. Toleration of increasing doses of the drug does develop through both metabolic and pharmacodynamic mechanisms, but the most important aspect of this is the mild level of cross-tolerance to alcohol that can be demonstrated.[1,8,15]

7.1.1.3.2. Dependence

There is some debate as to whether there is an actual withdrawal syndrome from marijuana. If it does occur, the strength probably parallels the amount and length of exposure to the drug and consists of nausea, lowered appetite, mild anxiety, and insomnia.[8,15,16] It is possible, however, that with higher doses a syndrome resembling mild opiate withdrawal may be noted.[15]

7.1.2. Epidemiology and Pattern of Abuse

The usual distinction made in this text between medical use and "street" use is not as relevant to marijuana as it is to many other drugs. While, some medical use of this drug is being evaluated, all but an infinitesimal amount of use of THC-containing substances takes place in illegal settings.

Marijuana is used as a "recreational" drug at all strata of society, reaching into all job levels and ages, although the predominant use is among younger people. It has been tried by some 36,000,000 Americans,[8] with over 50% of people age 18–25 reporting some use,[8] 20% using it two or more times a week, and 8% daily.[4] One in five adults reports having used marijuana at some time, and 20% of 18- to 25-year-olds report having tried hashish.[8]

Use of these drugs usually begins early, with 6% of 12- to 14-year-olds having tried marijuana. Once begun, the usual pattern is smoking several times a week to several times a month. Those individuals most likely to use marijuana on a frequent basis tend to demonstrate other life problems, including delinquency and polydrug misuse.[17]

7.1.3. Medical Uses

The purported medicinal properties of THC resulted in wide use until legislation limiting its availability was introduced shortly after the turn of the century.[1] The drug was listed in the *Pharmacopeia* until the 1930s as having antibacterial activity, decreasing intraocular pressure, decreasing perception of pain, helping in the treatment of asthma, containing anticonvulsant properti. (although recent evidence disputes this[12]), increasing appetite, and helping with general morale.[1,16] Currently, THC is being used experimentally for glaucoma which has been otherwise resistant to therapy[18] and for terminal cancer.

7.1.4. Establishing the Diagnosis

Recognizing whether psychiatric and medical problems are associated with marijuana and hashish use requires knowledge of the drug and an adequate history. While THC is thought to exacerbate depression and intensify any preexisting psychosis,[19] there are no known pathognomonic physical signs and no available laboratory tests to help. Again, the key is having a high index of suspicion.

7.2. EMERGENCY PROBLEMS

The vast majority of individuals presenting with marijuana-related problems show either panic or toxic reactions.[11] These involve high levels of anxiety and/or confusion.

7.2.1. Panic Reaction (See Sections 1.6.1., 5.2.1., 8.2.1., and 12.2.)

7.2.1.1. The Clinical Picture

This is a classic drug-induced panic, lasting at most five to eight hours.[3] The clinical picture includes an exaggeration of the usual marijuana effects, which commonly are perceived as threatening by the naive or inexperienced user.[8] The feeling of anxiety, the fear of losing control or going crazy, and the fear of physical illness can be seen in individuals with no preexisting psychopathology as well as in those demonstrating a history of erratic or maladaptive behavior.[20]

7.2.1.2. Treatment

Treatment is predicated on careful diagnosis, ruling out the involvement of other drugs and preexisting psychopathology,[19] and gentle reassurance.

1. A physical examination is necessary to rule out signs of other drugs of intoxication and preexisting medical disorders. It is advisable to draw bloods (10 ml) or collect urine (50 ml) for a toxicology screen.

2. A quick history should establish the dose taken and the individual's prior experience with the drug.

3. The individual should be reassured that his problems will clear within the next four to eight hours.

4. It helps to place the patient in a quiet room, constantly reassuring him, and allowing friends to help "talk him down."[2,20]

5. The level of intoxication may fluctuate over the next five hours or so, as active drug is released from the tissues.

6. No specific type of drug should be used to treat every panic reaction. If, however, the anxiety cannot be controlled in any other manner, the drugs of choice would be antianxiety medications, such as chlordiazepoxide (Librium), 10–50 mg orally which may be repeated in an hour, if needed.

7. Considering the persistence of THC metabolites in the body, patients should be warned that they may experience some mild feelings of drug intoxication over the next two to four days.

8. If the reaction is unusually intense, the patient as well as the family should be advised to seek evaluation for the possibility of preexist-

ing psychopathology. Referral to a physician or a health care practitioner experienced with drug problems is best.

7.2.2. Flashbacks (See Sections 1.6.2., and 8.2.2.)

7.2.2.1. The Clinical Picture

Flashbacks involve the spontaneous recurrence of feelings and perceptions experienced in the intoxicated state. They are classically seen for marijuana and hallucinogens,[3,8] in both frequent and infrequent users.

The clinical picture involves a change in time sense or a feeling of slowed thinking, generally at a lower level of intensity than that experienced when high. Because flashbacks tend to be time-limited (usually lasting only minutes), the major difficulty comes if the individual panics, fearing brain damage. It has also been reported that marijuana may "induce" flashbacks in individuals who have taken hallucinogens in the past.[11] In rare instances, the symptoms may be "chronic" or persistent, but this is so unusual that the presence of additional neurological or psychiatric disorders should be evaluated.

7.2.2.2. Treatment

Treatment of a flashback is simple reassurance, following all of the steps outlined in the treatment of the panic reaction (as outlined above).

7.2.3. Toxic Reactions (See Section 1.6.3.)

7.2.3.1. Clinical Picture

When an individual takes a high level of marijuana, toxic reactions can occur but are usually characterized by an OBS and/or paranoia as discussed in Sections 7.2.4., and 7.2.5. The relatively low potency of marijuana and the lack of availability of more toxic forms, such as ganja, in the United States combine to make this an infrequent problem.[8] Dangerous overdose is very rare for the cannabinols, even hashish.[15]

7.2.3.2. Treatment

Treatment is identicial to that outlined for panic reactions (Section 7.2.1.). The approach involves offering good general support and reassurance and allowing the passage of time in a room with no excessive external stimuli. It is best to treat this disorder symptomatically, avoiding the administration of other drugs.

7.2.4. Psychosis (See Sections 1.6.4., and 8.2.4.)

A *temporary* psychotic state, characterized by paranoia and hallucinations without confusion, can be seen with marijuana, but there is no evidence that it results in permanent mental impairment.

7.2.4.1. The Clinical Pictures

The temporary paranoid state accompanied by visual hallucinations is probably a reaction to excessive doses of the drug.[9,21] Retrospective studies indicate bizarre behavior, violence, and panic in some heavy users in India, but this reaction appears to be temporary.[22]

If a frankly psychotic state does not clear within hours to days, the patient generally has a prior psychiatric disorder, as marijuana probably worsens prior psychotic problems.[23] In addition, I have seen a number of people who had clear evidence of prior depressions or who demonstrated a prior psychotic picture, who complained that their present symptoms were caused by marijuana. In taking a history from the individual and relatives, the preexisting illness became obvious, and in many instances the history of drug ingestion was a delusion.

Anecdotal reports indicate the development of apathy, decreased self-awareness, impaired social judgment, slow thinking, and a decrease in goal-directed drives in chronic THC users.[1,3,24] However, these reports do not address any changes in personality occurring *prior to* marijuana use, perhaps predisposing users to heavy doses of the drug. An equally acceptable explanation is that individuals who are becoming apathetic and withdrawing from competition and from society in general also find chronic use of marijuana attractive. However, while no cognitive deficits have been objectively demonstrated in chronic users,[7,25] it is possible (although unlikely) that an *amotivational syndrome* exists where the person loses interest in tasks and accomplishments.

7.2.4.2. Treatment

It is imperative that a history of prior psychiatric problems be obtained in all individuals presenting with what appears to be a marijuana-induced psychosis.[11] The underlying prior psychiatric diagnosis (e.g., affective disorder or schizophrenia, as described by Woodruff *et al.*[26]) is the most important factor to be addressed in treatment.

1. If the individual is out of contact with reality, a short-term hospitalization can keep him out of trouble until the psychosis clears.

2. Understanding and reassurance is the cornerstone of treatment of these disorders. The individual should be told that his problem is tem-

porary, and attempts should be made to help him with reality testing by, for example, giving him insight into his hallucinations and delusions.

3. Antipsychotic medication can be initiated on a short-term basis if behavior control is absolutely necessary. You might use haloperidol (Haldol) at approximately 5 mg per day in divided doses (rarely up to 20 mg daily), or chlorpromazine (Thorazine) at 25–50 mg IM or 50 to 150 mg PO.

4. Anyone demonstrating a grossly psychotic reaction that lasts more than a day should be carefully evaluated for other major psychiatric disorders. The most frequent will probably be schizophrenia or affective disorder as described in Woodruff et al.[26]

7.2.5. Organic Brain Syndrome (See Section 1.6.5.)

7.2.5.1. The Clinical Pictures

1. Temporary clouding of mental processes, consisting of impaired and dull thinking, decreased memory, and decreased concentration, can occur with marijuana and hashish. This is really a toxic reaction and clears fairly rapidly.[27]

2. More startling is a report of cerebral ventricular dilatation (which may indicate cerebral hemisphere shrinkage) in 10 heavy drug users whose major drug was marijuana[28]—but all attempts to replicate these findings have failed.[8] To date, no convincing evidence of permanent decreased brain functioning in heavy users of THC substances has been shown.[29,30]

7.2.5.2. Treatment

The temporary type of clinical picture and the relatively mild level of impairment make the center of treatment careful observation and reassurance. Treatment involves the same steps outlined for the panic reaction in Section 7.2.1.2.

7.2.6. Withdrawal

It is not certain whether any form of withdrawal of clinical significance occurs with marijuana and hashish. If symptoms develop the picture can be expected to be limited and to clear with time alone.

7.2.7. Medical Problems

No drug can be taken into the body with complete safety. The medical disorders associated with frequent use of marijuana tend to be relatively mild and transient; but recognizing the purely recreational nature of this drug, it is hard to justify its use even if the possibility of serious medical complications is remote. Despite the long history of use of marijuana, it has been only in recent years that serious research has been carried out into the possible medical consequences.

The risk of adverse consequences, of course, increases with increasing amount, frequency of intake, and length of exposure to these drugs. Some of the more important areas of possible damage are presented below, primarily to help you in answering questions from patients and their relatives.

7.2.7.1. Effect on the Lungs[4,7,13]

1. Marijuana and other inhaled compounds are irritating and produce a bronchitis that usually disappears with discontinuation of drug use.

2. Although acute administration of marijuana causes dilatation of the bronchial tree, chronic administration is thought to cause constriction, with a resulting asthmalike syndrome.

3. Chronic use of any substance that irritates the lungs can cause temporary or permanent destruction of lung architecture, and there is evidence for a decreased vital capacity in chronic smokers—even healthy young men.[7]

4. While it is extremely difficult to document accurately, there is some evidence that heavy marijuana smokers have increased rates of precancerous lung lesions.

7.2.7.2. Nose and Throat

A chronic inflammation of the sinuses (sinusitis) has been reported in heavy smokers of marijuana. There is also the possibility (without any good direct evidence) that heavy marijuana smokers have the same increased risk for cancers of the head and neck as heavy tobacco smokers.

7.2.7.3. Cardiovascular System

Marijuana produces an increased heart rate and a decreased strength of heart contractions. This is dangerous for heart patients, as there is an associated decrease in oxygen delivery to heart muscle and a decrease in the amount of exercise an individual can tolerate before the onset of heart pain or angina.[14]

7.2.7.4. Immunity

Some research indicates that lymphocytes are sensitive to THC which decreases their ability to carry out the usual immune responses. It has not yet been determined whether this impairment results in a clinically significant increase in infections in marijuana users.

7.2.7.5. Reproduction

THC has been demonstrated to impair sperm production in heavy users[4] and has been associated with an increased rate of chromosomal breakage. The clinical importance of these findings has not been demonstrated.

7.2.7.6. Hormone Levels

Decreased levels of various hormones, including testosterone, have been demonstrated in heavy marijuana smokers,[21] but these abnormalities appear to be temporary and are usually seen only after three weeks of regular use. It is also possible that growth-hormone production is decreased in heavy marijuana smokers, but the clinical significance of this finding has not been established.

7.2.7.7. The Brain

CNS problems have been briefly discussed above in Sections 7.2.3., and 7.2.5. Heavy marijuana smokers may show changes in EEG tracings that may last for three months or more after chronic use.[4] THC has also been noted to act on the septal area of the limbic system—an area important in the control of emotions. These findings may have some importance for brain disease, especially in adolescents.

7.2.7.8. Allergies

Some individuals demonstrate allergic reactions to marijuana.[31] These are usually transient and probably of little clinical significance.

7.2.7.9. Diabetes

The use of marijuana by diabetics can result in a potentially life-threatening alteration in the body's acid-base metabolism, ketoacidosis.[32]

Thus, THC is not a benign drug and individuals choosing to use this substance should recognize the potential dangers. On the other hand, in educating people about THC, it is important to portray the dangers accurately and avoid scare tactics that might lead the young user to mistrust all information about the drug.

7.2.8. Other Emergency Problems

7.2.8.1. Accidents

One of the greatest known dangers of marijuana is accidents as a consequence of the decreased judgment, the impaired time and distance estimation, and the impaired motor performance that follow use. These problems are similar to the effects of alcohol, and it appears that the two substances may potentiate each other.[1,7] Thus, there is impressive evidence that marijuana smoking significantly decreases automobile-driving ability and impairs the faculties necessary to fly airplanes.[33] With wider use of this drug, one can expect greater loss of property and lives from driving under the influence of marijuana and related substances.

7.2.8.2. Precipitation of Use of Other Drugs

A brief notation is necessary to deal with public fears that the use of marijuana is the first step on the road to more dangerous drugs, such as heroin. Such exaggerated reports have been prevalent since the 1920s and have done little to establish the credibility of individuals teaching that TCH-containing substances have some real dangers.

The data in this area are very complex, as marijuana (as well as tobacco and alcohol) is frequently one of the first drugs taken by those who go on to the use of stimulants, depressants, or heroin.[34] There is, however, no convincing evidence that marijuana plays a role in "causing" the use of more potent substances. Rather, it is likely that individuals with characteristics leading them to use drugs like heroin also tend to use marijuana (and alcohol, caffeine, etc.).

REFERENCES

1. Jaffe, J. H. Drug addiction and drug abuse. In L. S. Goodman & A. Gilman (Eds.), *The Pharmacological Basis of Therapeutics*, 5th Ed. New York: Macmillan, 1975, pp. 284–324.
2. Liskow, B. Marijuana deterioration. *Journal of the American Medical Association. 214:*1709, Nov. 30, 1970.
3. Talbott, J. A. The emergency management of marijuana psychosis. In P. G. Bourne (Ed.), *A Treatment Manual for Acute Drug Abuse Emergencies*. Washington, D.C.: U.S. Government Printing Office, 1974, pp. 83–87.
4. Nahas, G. Biomedical aspects of cannabis usage. *Bulletin on Narcotics.* 24(2):13–27, 1977.
5. Lemberger, L., & Rubin, A. The physiologic disposition of marihuana in man. *Life Sciences.* 17:1637–1642, 1975.
6. Stillman, R., Galanter, M., & Lemberger, L. Tetrahydrocannabinol (THC): Metabolism and subjective effects. *Life Sciences.* 19:569–576, 1976.
7. Mendelson, J. H., Rossi, A. M., & Meyer, R. E. *The Use of Marihuana: A Psychological and Physiological Inquiry.* New York: Plenum Press, 1974.

8. Secretary of Health, Education, and Welfare. *Marijuana and Health*. Sixth Annual Report to the U.S. Congress. Rockville, Md.: National Institute on Drug Abuse, 1976.

9. Galanter, M., Stillman, R., Wyatt, R. J., *et al.* Marihuana and Social Behavior. A controlled study. *Archives of General Psychiatry. 30*:518–521, 1974.

10. Weil, A. T., Zinberg, N. E., & Nelsen, J. M. Clinical and psychological effects of marihuana in man. *Science. 162*:1234–1242, 1968.

11. Weil, A. T. Adverse reactions to marihuana. Classification and suggested treatment. *New England Journal of Medicine. 282*(18):997–1000, 1970.

12. Feeney, D. M. Marihuana and epilepsy. *Science. 197*:1301–1302, 1977.

13. Cohen, S., & Stillman, R. C. *The Therapeutic Potential of Marihuana*. New York: Plenum Medical Book Company, 1976.

14. Gottschalk, L. A., Aronow, W. S., & Prakash, R. Effect of marijuana and placebo-marijuana smoking of psychological state and on psychophysiological cardiovascular functioning in anginal patients. *Biological Psychiatry. 12*(2):255–266, 1977.

15. Kaymakcalan, S. Potential dangers of cannabis. *International Journal of the Addictions. 10*(14):721–735, 1975.

16. Cohen, S. Marihuana: Does it have medical usefulness? *Drug Abuse and Alcoholism Newsletter. 5*(10), 1976.

17. Halikas, J. A., Goodwin, D. W., & Guze, S. B. Marihuana use and psychiatric illness. *Archives of General Psychiatry. 27*:162–165, 1972.

18. Hepler, R. S., & Petrus, R. Experiences with administration of marihuana to glaucoma patients. In S. Cohen & R. C. Stillman (Eds.), *The Therapeutic Potential of Marihuana*. New York: Plenum Medical Book Company, 1976, pp. 63–76.

19. Treffert, D. A. Marihuana use in schizophrenia: A clear hazard. Presented at the 130th Annual Meeting of the American Psychiatric Assocation, Toronto, Ontario, Canada, May 5, 1977.

20. Pillard, R. C. Marihuana. *New England Journal of Medicine. 283*(6):292–304, 1970.

21. Naditch, M. P. Acute adverse reactions to psychoactive drugs. *Journal of Abnormal Psychology. 83*:394–403, 1974.

22. Halikas, J. A. Marijuana use and psychiatric illness. In L. L. Miller (Ed.), *Marijuana: Effects on Human Behavior*. New York: Academic Press, 1974, pp. 265–302.

23. Ablon, S. L., & Goodwin, F. K. High frequency of dysphoric reactions of tetrahydrocannabinol among depressed patients. *American Journal of Psychiatry. 131*(4):448–453, 1974.

24. Kolansky, H., & Moore, W. T. Marihuana, can it hurt you? *Journal of the American Medical Association. 232*(9):923–924, 1975.

25. Brill, N. Q., & Christie, R. L. Marihuana use and psychosocial adaptation. Follow-up study of a collegiate population. *Archives of General Psychiatry. 31*:713–719, 1974.

26. Woodruff, R. A., Goodwin, D. W., & Guze, S. B. *Psychiatric Diagnosis*. New York: Oxford University Press, 1974.

27. Meyer, R. E. Psychiatric consequences of marijuana use. In J. R. Tinklenberg (Ed.), *Marijuana and Health Hazards*. New York: Academic Press, 1975, pp. 133–152.

28. Campbell, A. M. G., Evans, M., Thomason, J. L. G., *et al.* Cerebral atrophy in young canabis smokers. *Lancet II:* 1219–1224, 1971.

29. Grant, I., & Mohns, L. Chronic cerebral effects of alcohol and drug abuse. *International Journal of the Addictions. 10*(5):883–920, 1975.

30. Stefanis, C., Laikos, A., Boulougouris, J., *et al.* Chronic hashish use and mental disorder. *American Journal of Psychiatry.* 133(2):225–227, 1976.

31. Liskow, B., Liss, J. L., & Parker, C. W. Allergy to marihuana. *Annals of Internal Medicine.* 75:571–574, 1971.

32. Bier, M. M., & Steahly, L. P. Emergency treatment of marihuana complicating diabetes. In P. G. Bourne (Ed.), *A Treatment Manual for Acute Drug Abuse Emergencies.* Washington, D.C.: U.S. Government Printing Office, 1974, pp. 88–94.

33. Janowsky, D. S., Meacham, M. P., Blaine, J. D., *et al.* Simulated flying performance after marihuana intoxication. *Aviation, Space, and Environmental Medicine.* Feb. 1976, pp. 124–128.

34. Kandel, D. Stages in adolescent involvement in drug use. *Science.* 190:912–914, 1975.

CHAPTER 8

The Hallucinogens, PCP, and Related Drugs

8.1. INTRODUCTION

Both marijuana and the hallucinogens produce a change in the level of consciousness, and both are capable of inducing hallucinations. However, in the usual doses taken, the predominant effect of cannabis is to alter the "feeling state" without frank hallucinations, whereas the drugs discussed in this chapter produce abnormal sensory inputs of a predominantly visual nature (illusions or hallucinations) even at low doses.

This chapter covers a variety of substances, as shown in Table 8.1. These drugs are structurally similar; many resemble amphetamine; some (e.g., LSD) are synthetic, while others are plant products of cacti (e.g.,

Table 8.1
Hallucinogenic Drugs[23]

Indolealkylamines
LSD
Psilocybin
Psilocyn
Dimethyltryptamine (DMT)
Diethyltryptamine (DET)
Phenylethylamines
Mescaline (peyote)
Phenylisopropylamines
2,5-dimethoxy-4-methyl-amphetamine (DOM or STP)
Related drugs
Phencyclidine (PCP)
Nutmeg
Morning glory seeds
Catnip
Nitrous oxide
Amyl or Butyl Nitrite

peyote or mescaline) and fungi (e.g., psilocybin). Hallucinogens have no medical uses in which their assets are known to outweigh their liabilities.[1]

The hallucinogens are by no means new substances. They have been used as part of religious ceremonies and at social gatherings by native Americans for over 2,000 years[2] and are still utilized by some native groups.[3,4]

8.1.1. Pharmacology

All drugs of this class are well absorbed orally, exert effects at relatively low doses, and have adrenergic (e.g., adrenalinelike) properties. Lysergic acid diethylamide (LSD) is the prototype, and the generalizations given for this drug can be assumed to hold for the other drugs as well, unless noted in the text.

The exact mechanism of action of these substances is not known, but much study has centered on their structural similarities to brain transmitters.[5] The term *psychotomimetic* has also been used, implying a possible relationship between the hallucinogen psychoses and schizophrenia. The visual hallucinations and the strong emotional state seen with these substances, however, do not resemble the auditory hallucinations accompanied by a flat (or unchanging) affect seen in schizophrenics.

The hallucinogens differ in length of action, with the "high" from LSD lasting as long as 6–12 hours and most others acting for 2–4 hours. The rate of metabolism tends, of course, to parallel the length of action, with the half-life for LSD being approximately 3 hours.[6]

8.1.1.1. Predominant Effects

The state induced by these substances (also called *psychedelic drugs*) includes an increased awareness of sensory input, a subjective feeling of enhanced mental activity, a perception of usual environmental stimuli as novel events, altered body images,[7] a turning of thoughts inward, and a decreased ability to tell the difference between oneself and one's surroundings.[6] This group of related drugs tends to produce adrenalinelike or adrenergic effects in addition to hallucinations. Thus, the intoxicated individual usually exhibits dilated pupils, a flushed face, a fine tremor,[8] increased blood pressure, elevations in blood sugar,[8] and an increase in body temperature.[9,10]

8.1.1.2. Tolerance and Dependence

8.1.1.2.1. Tolerance

Toleration of larger and larger doses develops rapidly after as little as three or four days at one dose per day and disappears within four days to a week after stopping use. Cross-tolerance exists between most of the hallucinogens, including LSD, mescaline, and psilocybin; but this cross-tolerance does not appear to extend to marijuana.[4,11]

8.1.1.2.2. Dependence

There is no known clinically significant withdrawal syndrome with the hallucinogens.

8.1.1.3. Specific Drugs

Thus far in this text, most of the drugs described are readily available on the street and are usually the drugs the seller advertises them to be (a notable exception has been the virtual nonexistence of pure THC). This, however, is *not* the case for the hallucinogens. Studies have demonstrated that, while 87% of LSD samples are pure, as high as 95% of mescaline or peyote units contain either no drug, phencyclidine (PCP—see Section 8.3.), or LSD; and similar figures probably exist for the other hallucinogens.[12] In addition, even those samples that actually contain the noted substance usually also contain an adulterant such as amphetamines.[8,13] Thus, it is *not* safe to assume that one can predict the reaction just by knowing what substance the individual *thinks* he is taking.

Briefly, the more common drugs include:

8.1.1.3.1. LSD

This is a very potent drug that produces frank hallucinations at doses as low as 20–35 μg, with the usual street dose ranging from 50 to 300 μg.[4] At doses as low as 0.5–2.0 μg/kg, the individual experiences dizziness, weakness, and a series of physiological changes that are replaced by euphoria and hallucinations lasting from 4 to 12 hours. The actual "high" depends upon the dose, the individual's emotional set, the environment, prior drug experiences, and psychiatric history.

LSD can be purchased as a powder, a solution, a capsule or a pill. The colorless, tasteless substance is also sold dissolved on sugar cubes or pieces of blotter. While the drug is usually taken orally, it has been known to be administered subcutaneously (SQ) or intravenously (IV). LSD may be placed on tobacco and smoked, but the intoxication obtained by this method is usually quite mild.[4]

8.1.1.3.2. Mescaline or Peyote

The hard, dried brown buttons of the peyote cactus contain mescaline, the second most widely used hallucinogen.[4] Mescaline effects have a slower onset than those of LSD and are frequently accompanied by unpleasant side effects, such as nausea and vomiting. The hallucinations usually last 1–2 hours after a usual dose of 300–500 mg.

8.1.1.3.3. Psilocybin

Psilocybin is obtained from mushrooms, many of which grow wild in the United States, with resulting hallucinations similar to those noted for LSD and mescaline. It is usually taken by mouth and has a rapid onset with effects demonstrated within 15 minutes after a 4–8 mg dose. Reactions peak at about 90 minutes and begin to wane at 2–3 hours, but they do not disappear for 5–6 hours. Larger doses tend to produce longer periods of intoxication.[4]

8.1.1.3.4. DOM or STP

This is a synthetic hallucinogen, bearing a structural resemblance to both amphetamine and mescaline and resembling LSD in its effects.[4] The usual dose is 5 or more mg; thus, the drug is between 50 and 100 times less potent than LSD. The onset of effects is usually within 1 hour of ingestion and peak effects occur at 3–5 hours, disappearing by 7 or 8 hours.[4] The physiological changes are adrenalinelike, paralleling those of LSD. It may be that the effects of this substance are intensified following the administration of chlorpromazine (Thorazine).[4]

8.1.2. Epidemiology and Patterns of Abuse

The hallucinogens were, along with marijuana, the first of the "middle-class" street drugs to cause public concern in the 1960s. While it is impossible to be certain of the extent of abuse, studies of the street culture, as well as emergency room admissions, indicate a peak prevalence in 1966–1967, with a subsequent leveling off and decline.[4,9] Hallucinogens remain in general use but have been somewhat replaced in popularity by the stimulants and depressants.

These drugs are probably used on an occasional basis by approximately 20% of the youth population.[14] With the exception of native Americans' utilizing peyote as part of religious ceremonies, the "ritual" use of hallucinogens by various subcultural groups has diminished.

8.2. EMERGENCY PROBLEMS FOR LSD-TYPE DRUGS

The most common hallucinogen-related difficulties seen in emergency rooms are panic reactions, flashbacks, and toxic reactions. In addition, temporary psychoses (actually, probably toxic reactions) and a limited number of medical problems have been noted and need to be discussed.

8.2.1. Panic Reaction (See Sections 1.6.1., 5.2.1., 7.2.1., and 12.2.)

8.2.1.1. Clinical Picture

Because these drugs cause both stimulation and hallucinations at relatively low doses, it is not surprising that the most common problem for hallucinogens seen in emergency room settings is the high level of anxiety and fear that characterize the panic reaction.[6] In the panic state, the individual is highly stimulated, frightened, hallucinating, and usually fearful of losing his mind. This is one example of a "bad trip," the other being the toxic reaction seen in individuals who have taken higher than the usual clinical dosages (see Section 8.2.3.).

Panic reactions are usually found only in people with limited prior exposure to hallucinogens. The emotional discomfort tends to last for the length of action of the drug, for example, up to 12 hours for LSD and closer to 2–4 hours for mescaline and peyote.

8.2.1.2. Treatment

1. Therapy is based on reassurance[6] by explaining the process of a panic reaction to the individual and reassuring him that he will totally recover.

2. For added comfort, care should be given if possible in the presence of friends or family members.[15]

3. It is important that a supportive, nonthreatening environment be established where constant verbal contact can be maintained.[16]

4. Hospitalization is not usually needed if a temporary, quiet, safe atmosphere can be arranged.[17]

5. Medications are usually *not* needed. However, if it is impossible to control the patient otherwise, most authors suggest the use of an antianxiety drug such as:

    a. Diazepam (Valium), 10–30 mg orally, repeated in 1–2 hours as needed,[9] or

    b. Chlordiazepoxide (Librium) in doses of 10–50 mg orally which may be repeated in 1–2 hours.[18]

    c. Do not use chlorpromazine (Thorazine) or any other antipsychotic drug because of the possibility that the hallucinogen might be STP (see Section 8.1.1.3.4.) or that the antipsychotics might increase any anticholinergic effects of adulterants in the ingested drug.[16]

6. It is important to obtain a clear history of drug misuse and prior psychiatric disorders and to establish a differential diagnosis, particularly ruling out mania and schizophrenia.[16,19]

7. It is suggested that a follow-up visit be arranged to help the individual deal with his drug-taking problems and to rule out any major coexisting psychiatric disorder.[16]

8.2.2. Flashbacks (See Section 1.6.2., and 7.2.2.)

8.2.2.1. Clinical Picture

This relatively *benign* condition usually comes to the attention of the health care practitioner because an individual becomes concerned that the recurrence of drug effects represents permanent brain damage.[20] In the midst of such a state, he may demonstrate sadness, anxiety, or even paranoia, which may recur periodically for days to weeks after taking the drug.[21] It is thought that this recurrence of hallucinogen effects represents, in part, residual drug metabolites and may be set off by taking a milder drug such as marijuana or by an acute crisis.

The person usually notes a feeling of euphoria and detachment, which is frequently associated with visual illusions (actual sensory inputs that are misinterpreted by the individual) lasting several minutes to hours.[9] The hallucinations are usually lights or geometric figures seen out of the corner of the eye, often when entering darkness or just before falling asleep, or a trail of light following a moving object. Only rarely do they interfere with an individual's ability to function. Other types of flashbacks, including isolated feelings of depersonalization or a recurrence of distressing emotional reactions experienced while under the drug effects, can also occur.[9] The incidence of these reactions is not known, but they have been estimated to occur in as high as 5% of users.[9]

8.2.2.2. Treatment

Therapy for the self-limited picture is relatively simple:[9]

1. Care is based on reassurance that the syndrome will gradually decrease in intensity and disappear.

2. The subject should be educated about the course and the probable causes (e.g., residual drug) for the flashback.

3. It is important that all other medications, especially marijuana, antihistamines, and stimulants, be avoided.[8]

4. If medication is needed to relax the individual during the experience (I usually choose to use no medication), use diazepam (Valium) in doses of 10–20 mg orally, repeated at 5-mg doses if the flashback recurs[9] or comparable oral doses of chlordiazepoxide (e.g., 10–30 mg).

5. As is true in any drug related disorder, in an emergency situation it is important to consider the possibility that the problem is a reflection of a preexisting psychiatric disorder and not really a flashback. Therefore, a careful *history of prior psychiatric problems and a family history of psychiatric illness* (which may indicate a propensity toward illness for this individual) must be taken.

8.2.3. Toxic Reactions (See Sections 2.2.3., 5.2.3., 6.2.3., and 12.4.)

8.2.3.1. The Clinical Picture

8.2.3.1.1. History

The usual toxic reaction consists of the rapid onset (over minutes to hours) of a loss of contact with reality and the physical symptoms described below in an individual taking a hallucinogen. The markedly disturbed behavior usually leads friends or relatives to bring the patient in for care.

8.2.3.1.2. Physical Signs and Symptoms

While the psychological state dominates the picture for the average patient, abnormalities in vital signs that are consistent with the state of anxiety and panic are also seen. These include palpitations, increases in blood pressure and temperature, perspiration, and possibly blurred vision. Very high levels of overdose may include exceedingly high body temperatures (greater than 103°F orally), shock, and convulsions.[23,24]

8.2.3.1.3. Psychological State

This is an exaggeration of the effects of a panic reaction. The individual, frequently an experienced user, has taken a higher than usual dose of the drug, with a resulting high anxiety state along with frank hallucinations and loss of contact with reality.[22] Depersonalization, paranoia, and confusion are often demonstrated.[9] The clinical picture diminishes as the drug is metabolized, but the symptoms tend to wax and wane over the subsequent 8–24 hours.[23]

8.2.3.1.4. Relevant Laboratory Tests

There are no specific laboratory tests to be noted except for the possible use of a toxicologic screen (10 ml of blood or 50 ml of urine). It is important to monitor vital signs, especially blood pressures and body temperature. If signs of organicity are present, it is necessary to rule out ancillary causes, including head trauma and infection.

8.2.3.2. Treatment (See Sections 2.2.3.2., 5.2.3.2., and 6.2.3.2.)

1. Although quite rare, the overdose may involve markedly elevated drug levels and the patient may present with convulsions or hyperthermia. The treatment steps for any life-threatening drug emergency must be carried out.[24] These include:

    a. Careful observation of vital signs
    b. Establishing an airway
    c. Treatment of convulsions with anticonvulsants and a slow injection of diazepam (5–20 mg IV), if needed (see Section 5.2.3.2.)
    d. The use of ice baths or a hypothermic blanket
    e. Cardiac monitoring, support of blood pressure by medications, if needed (see Section 6.2.3.2., and 12.4.3.) etc.

2. For the usual patient with relatively stable vital signs, a rapid physical examination, including a neurological evaluation, should be carried out. Vital signs should be monitored for at least 24 hours.[23]

3. It is important to gain the patient's confidence with an understanding but firm approach. Consistent verbal contact and reality-orienting cues must be given, generally for up to 24 hours.

4. The rapid absorption of most of these drugs would indicate that gastric lavage is of little use and may only serve to frighten the patient.[23]

5. Once again, I prefer to avoid medication, but when necessary I usually fall back on:

    a. Diazepam (Valium) 15–30 mg orally repeating 5–20 mg every four hours as needed
    b. *Or* Chlordiazepoxide (Librium) at 10–50 mg orally, followed by up to 25–50 mg every four hours as needed
    c. *Avoid* chlorpromazine (Thorazine) or any other antipsychotic drug

6. If the clinical problem does not clear within 24 hours, suspect that the drug ingested was STP (which might last for several days to two weeks) or PCP, as discussed in Sections 8.1.1.3.4., and 8.3. Treatment in this situation is very similar to that outlined above; however, vital signs must be carefully monitored.

8.2.4. Psychosis (See Sections 1.6.4., 5.2.4., and 7.2.4.)

8.2.4.1. Clinical Picture

In my experience, hallucinogen-induced psychoses (most often marked by visual hallucinations) clear within hours to days and (for STP) certainly within a matter of weeks. The literature substantiates that those rare individuals for whom the psychosis does not clear have a preexisting psychiatric problem, usually mania, schizophrenia, or a psychotic depression. The causes of hallucinogen psychoses are difficult to study and are frequently complicated by multiple-drug use.[25] As would be expected, the psychotic syndrome has a wide variety of presentations, including depression, panic, uncontrolled hallucinations, and/or intensification or a preexisting paranoid picture.[6,26]

One special area for consideration is a crime committed under the apparent influence of LSD or other hallucinogens. If the criminal act is a well-thought-out, goal-oriented one, and especially if criminal behavior is consistent with the individual's prior experiences and activities, I would tend to discount the role played by LSD in the commission of the crime.[27]

8.2.4.2. Treatment

The actual treatment must depend upon the clinical picture.

1. If on reevaluation, one finds an intense panic or toxic reaction, the treatment is as described in Sections 8.2.1.2., and 8.2.3.2.

2. In an individual with a preexisting affective disorder, obvious schizophrenia, etc., emergency treatment for a psychotic reaction resembles that outlined in Section 8.2.3.2., but the most important therapy is aimed at the specific psychiatric disorder.[19]

3. A drug-induced psychosis occurring in an individual without preexisting psychiatric disorder is treated with reassurance, education, and comfort in a manner similar to that outlined in Sections 8.2.1.2., and 8.2.3.2.[8] Hospitalization may be required if the loss of contact with reality is severe.

4. If the psychosis does not clear within 24 hours and no prior psychiatric disorder is apparent, it is imperative that the individual be carefully evaluated for any neurological damage, that a thorough physical examination and laboratory tests be carried out, and that the practitioner recognize the unusual nature of the syndrome. As with any atypical picture, treatment is symptomatic, requiring careful observation, good history-taking, and constant reevaluation for possible underlying pathological diagnoses. There is no set procedure in this instance, and antipsychotic drugs, if used, should be carefully monitored.

8.2.5. Organic Brain Syndrome (See Section 1.6.5.)

8.2.5.1. Clinical Picture

An organic picture can develop in the midst of a toxic reaction or a severe overdose, or it can be part of a drug-induced psychosis. Treatment of these syndromes has been outlined above in Section 8.2.4.2.

A second major concern is that prolonged exposure to these drugs may cause a decreased intellectual functioning and even an organic brain syndrome. People chronically taking hallucinogens have been noted to demonstrate a syndrome similar to the purported "amotivational syndrome" already discussed about marijuana in Section 7.2.4. It is extremely difficult to establish a "cause-and-effect" relationship, as persons likely to use these drugs regularly may have tended toward social withdrawal, lack of motivation, and even brain impairment before the drug use was begun. The problem of establishing cause and effect is even more acute when multiple substances are taken.

There is some evidence, however, of a decrease in abstract reasoning seen in heavy users,[6] but this has not been corroborated in all groups studied.[28] Brain damage should be considered in evaluation of any chronic abuser of hallucinogens, but the probability of clinically significant impairment is remote.

8.2.5.2. Treatment

The individual suffering possible organic brain damage from continued hallucinogen use should be dealt with symptomatically, including recommendation for abstinence from drugs and all other medications (including alcohol), reevaluation of degree of impairment over time, and vocational or educational rehabilitation, if appropriate.

8.2.6. Withdrawal

No clinically significant withdrawal picture is known for the hallucinogens.

8.2.7. Medical Problems

Evaluation of chronic users of hallucinogens has rarely demonstrated unique physiological impairment directly related to the drugs.[29,30] One area of great concern has been the possiblity of *chromosomal damage*.[3] While broken chromosomes have certainly been demonstrated with LSD-type drugs and birth abnormalities have been seen in offspring of mothers using hallucinogens (especially LSD in the first trimester), the nature of the relationship has not been established. Many substances (including aspirin) cause chromosomal breakage but have not been demonstrated to have definitely affected the fetus. Nonetheless, these are very potent substances, and there may be a danger of fetal abnormality when they are used by pregnant women.[31-33]

8.3. PHENCYCLIDINE (PCP) OR ANGEL DUST

8.3.1. Introduction

This drug was originally introduced as a general anesthetic agent. It has mostly disappeared from legal human use since the mid 1960s, although it is still used as a veterinarian anesthetic (Synalar or Sernylan) and is similar to an anesthetic used for the elderly and children (Ketalar).[35] Its advantage as an anesthetic agent was that it produced a disassociated state (feelings of unreality) with little lowering of respiratory rate or blood pressure.

The drug has become widely misused as a "hallucinogen" known on the street as *mist, hog, crystal, peace pill, tranq,* and animal tranquilizer. It is also a widely used adulterant or a substitute for other street substances such as LSD and THC.[36] PCP can be smoked (tending to cause a more mild intoxication) or ingested orally as well as injected intravenously or sprayed on other drugs such as marijuana.[36] The most usual routes of administration are smoking or oral ingestion.

8.3.2. Pharmacology

PCP is easily produced by amateur chemists in the kitchen. The crystaline powder effects the basic brain centers, probably through interference with the synaptic transmission between brain cells, perhaps creating an inbalance of catecholaminergic (or adrenalinelike) and cholinergic chemicals.

The drug is readily absorbed by mouth or through inhalation, and the onset of effects are rapid. The half-life is approximately one-half hour to an hour, but the length of action of the drug is longer as it seems to leave the blood and become bound to tissues. Metabolism is primarily in the liver with no known pharmacologic activities for metabolites.[36]

The major physiological effects at the usual doses are *sympathomimetic* in nature and include increases in blood pressure, heart rate, respiratory rate, and reflexes—the latter resulting in muscle rigidity. The drug also has *cholinergic* effects that include sweating, flushing, drooling, and pupillary constriction. *Cerebellar* effects may result in dizziness, uncoordination, slurred speech, and nystagmus.[37]

In relatively low doses (1–5 mg), the drug produces a floating feeling of euphoria and emotionality,[20] and higher doses (around 10 mg) are associated with a drunken state, numbness of the extremities, and illusions (misperceptions of defects). Even in this dose range there are reports of violent behavior, sometimes uncontrollable, accompanying intoxication. At larger doses the drug is associated with convulsions and a CNS-depressant-type death.

8.3.3. Epidemiology and Pattern of Abuse

The low cost and the ease with which PCP is manufactured by kitchen chemists have made this an increasingly popular drug. Approximately 20% of young people admit to some deliberate experimentaion with the drug,[37] and virtually all street samples of THC and a high percentage of hallucinogens actually contain PCP rather than the purported drug.

8.3.4. Emergency Situations for PCP

The rapid increase in the popularity of this drug has created a situation where PCP is involved in many types of emergency situations, few of which have been adequately studied.[38]

8.3.4.1. Panic Reaction (See Sections 1.6.1., 2.2.1., 5.2.1., 7.2.1., and 8.2.1.)

8.3.4.1.1. Clinical Picture

Although panic reactions have not been reported, as such, in the literature, they are to be expected considering PCP's sympathomimetic effects and its ability to produce illusions. These are probably of short duration, clearing within a matter of hours. However, it is advisable that the reader become acquainted with the course and treatment of panic reactions for stimulants, cannabinols, and the hallucinogens.

8.3.4.1.2. Treatment

Treatment of this condition is primarily symptomatic, allowing the patient to recover in a quiet setting. Should medications be needed (although I would caution against their use unless necessary) relatively low doses of oral antianxiety drugs will probably suffice (for example 10–20 mg of chlordiazepoxide [Librium] or 5–10 mg of diazepam [Valium]).[38]

8.3.4.2. Flashbacks (See Sections 7.2.2., and 8.2.2.)

Although not well documented, anecdotal reports indicate that a recurrence of the milder drug effects (e.g., feelings of unreality or mild sympathomimetic symptoms) probably occur.[39] These are generally not disturbing to the patient and are probably best treated with reassurance, although antianxiety drugs in doses similar to those listed for a panic reaction can be considered on a one- or, at most, two-dose schedule.

8.3.4.3. Toxic Reactions (See Sections 2.2.3., 5.2.3., 6.2.3., and 8.2.3.)

8.3.4.3.1. Clinical Picture

PCP has marked medical and psychological effects that vary greatly between individuals. The narrow dose range between the amount responsible for the usual intoxication and the dose responsible for a toxic reaction results in blurring the distinction between toxic, OBS, and panic reactions. Thus, in attempting to understand the clinical picture, it is important that all relevant sections of this chapter be read (see Sections 8.3.4.4., and 8.3.4.5.).

Medically, the toxic reaction consists of a combination of sympathetic and cholinergic overactivity that can be seen with doses as low as 5 mg. At lower dose ranges, symptoms include vertigo, skin flushing, nausea and vomiting, enhanced reflexes, a tremor, pupillary constriction (or no change in pupils), nystagmus and double vision, bilateral ptosis or drooping eyelids, increased blood pressure, as well as a dry mouth, drooling, etc. When higher doses are taken, in excess of 100 mg, symptoms can be life-threatening, including problems in decreased respirations, epileptic seizures, body rigidity, and coma. The combination of a comalike state, open eyes, decreased pain perception, temporary periods of excitation, and body rigiditiy should raise suspicion that a PCP toxic state is being observed.[38,39]

The psychological changes are characterized by a patient who is detached and may be unresponsive to external stimuli. However, an evanescent period of excitement and the hostility which can be seen with PCP may replace the comalike state. These are discussed in greater depth in Section 8.3.4.4.

8.3.4.3.2. Treatment

Treatment of this mixed state of serious physical and psychological impairment has not been well established. In dealing with patients, it is important to have some general understanding of treatment of toxic conditions as has been outlined in Sections 2.2.3., 4.2.3., 6.2.3., and 12.4. The necessary steps (not necessarily in any rigid order) are given to a patient who must be kept in as quiet an atmosphere as possible. These include:

1. Rule out all other possible causes of the obtunded condition and physical impairment. This will require an accurate neurological evaluation and drawing bloods (10 ml) or obtaining a urine sample (50 ml) for a toxicology screen.

2. Assistance to respiration may be required. Because of the high level of muscle rigidity which may be seen in a PCP intoxication state,

anesthetic levels of muscle relaxants may be required before intubation can be carried out.

3. Severe hypertension must be treated using agents like phentolamine (Regitine), giving an IV drip of 2–5 mg over 5–10 minutes, taking care not to lower the blood pressure too far.

4. When PCP was taken orally, gastric lavage should be considered, rinsing with saline until a clear return is seen. Of course, the precautions of using an inflatable cuff for the tracheal tube should be taken to avoid aspiration for patients in coma.

5. An IV should be begun using a large-gauge needle, as it may be necessary to replace fluid lost in the urine (along with 20 ml per hour of insensible loss).

6. Some authors have recommended diuresis using either furosemide (Lasix) at doses of 40–120 mg as often as necessary to maintain 250 ml or more of urine output per hour or through the use of excessive IV fluids, usually saline and water with glucose, to maintain a urinary output at the same level. However, I would caution against diuresis, as there is little proof that it is effective.[38,39]

All other general body supports should be maintained similar to those outlined in Sections, 2.2.3., and 12.4.

8.3.4.4. Psychosis

8.3.4.4.1. Clinical Picture

Consistently in this book, I have made the somewhat arbitrary distinction between hallucinations and/or delusions (a psychosis) occurring in the midst of a confused state (which is usually discussed either under the toxic state or an OBS) and the psychosis occurring with an otherwise clear mental status. With PCP, the state may fluctuate so that many individuals who develop a toxic reaction or an OBS will "improve" to the point of demonstrating a psychosis alone.[39,40]

The psychotic picture may consist of paranoia and/or manic behavior (for example grandiosity, hyperactivity, rapid thoughts and speech, etc.).[40,41] The patient may also show great emotional changes, including hostility accompanied by violent outbursts.[38,39] The degree and persistence of the psychosis appears to relate to the amount of drug ingested and, thus, the amount excreted in the urine[40] and can last from 24 hours to one month.

8.3.4.4.2. Treatment

The best treatment is probably to offer the patient a quiet, sheltered environment where his psychosis is not likely to lead to harm to either himself or those around him (i.e., a closed psychiatric ward). Treatment for medical and psychological problems should primarily be symptomatic, but I would recommend avoiding medications unless necessary. Should hostile outbursts occur, there is some general acceptance of the use of antianxiety drugs, for example, using either IM or oral diazepam (Valium) in doses up to 60 mg or comparable doses (perhaps up to 100 mg) of chlordiazepoxide (Librium). Adequate treatment of any psychotic state requires a careful evaluation to rule out any preexisting psychiatric disorders that might require treatment (for example, manic depressive disease or schizophrenia).

8.3.4.5. Organic Brain Syndrome

A state of confusion and/or decreased intellectual functioning is a part of the usual toxic reaction. Thus, the reader is referred to Section 8.3.4.3.

8.3.4.6. Withdrawal (See Section 1.6.6.)

Because of the structure of PCP, there may well be a withdrawal syndrome seen after chronic administration. This has, however, not yet been reported in the literature. Treatment would be symptomatic, perhaps requiring CNS depressants such as diazepam (Valium) to control symptoms.

8.3.4.7. Medical Complications

It is not yet known whether chronic misuse of these substances is associated with the failure of any major organ systems.

8.4. RELATED DRUGS

It is necessary to discuss separately a series of drugs that produce effects similar to the more common substances but whose structures do not allow for generalizations. The more exotic (and usually less potent) hallucinogens that require mention include *nutmeg, morning glory seeds, catnip, nitrous oxide,* and *amyl* or *butyl nitrite.*[34]

8.4.1. Nutmeg

The nutmeg plant can be ground up and either inhaled or ingested in large amounts to produce a change in consciousness.[6] The unpleasant side effects of these substances (including vomiting) limit their use to places where other drugs are not available, such as prisons.[6,42] The oral ingestion of two grated nutmeg pods will produce, after a latency of several hours, a feeling of heaviness in the arms and legs, a feeling of not being one's self (depersonalization), a feeling of unreality (derealization), and apprehension. Along with this reaction are physiological changes such as dry mouth, thirst, increased heart rate, and flushing.[6,42-44]

The specific mechanism of action of nutmeg is not known, but it is felt that it might inhibit prostaglandin. One of the side effects of chronic use may be constipation.[43]

The usual recovery from signs of intoxication occur within 24–48 hours. No specific treatment for the toxic reaction is needed. None of the other catagories of drug misuse problems is known to occur with nutmeg.

8.4.2. Morning Glory Seeds

The seeds of the more common varieties of morning glory flowers contain an LSD-related substance,[45,46] which, if ingested in high enough amounts, can produce a mild hallucinatory state. The usual effect of these substances, known as *heavenly blue* or *pearly gates*, is a change in self-awareness and visual hallucinations, which might be accompanied by paranoia. Taken intravenously, this drug can be very dangerous and has been shown to produce a lethal, shocklike state.[46]

Treatment of any panic, toxic, or potential psychotic reactions would follow that outlined for the hallucinogens as given in Sections 8.2.1.2., 8.2.3.2., and 8.2.4.2.

8.4.3. Catnip

This substance, derived from the plant *Nepeda cataria* (a member of the mint family), has a long history as a folk-medicine prescription for abdominal irregularities.[6] The plant contains a variety of substances, including tannin and atropinelike drugs. It can be obtained in pet stores and has been given to cats to make them appear happy, contented, and somewhat intoxicated. When used by humans, usually smoked, the intoxication can be quite similar to that from marijuana. Visual hallucinations, euphoria, and fairly rapid changes in mood are frequently associated with headaches, but these tend to clear rather quickly. There is no known treatment needed for the panic or toxic state that can be noted with the substance.

8.4.4. Nitrous Oxide (N₂O)

This is a relatively weak general anesthetic that is either used as an adjunct to other agents or given on its own by dentists and/or obstetricians.[6] Abuse of this inhalant tends to occur among profesisonals, but one recent case study indicated the abuse of N2O used as a propellant for canned whipped cream.[47] Use of the drug for a number of months on a daily basis can result in a paranoid psychotic state accompanied by confusion. As would be expected, this clears fairly rapidly when the drug use is stopped.[48]

8.4.5. Amyl or Butyl Nitrite

This drug, marketed under the name of Vaporole and also sold in "adult bookstores" as *Rush, Kick, Belt*, etc., dilates blood vessels and has been used in the treatment of angina, although it now has limited medical usefulness.[49] It is purported in the street culture that this drug causes a slight euphoria and flushing, may slow down time perception, and may postpone orgasm during sexual intercourse. There are few scientific data on these properties, and misuse of the drug is not now widespread. The most common clinical problems of intoxication are a toxic reaction and a panic reaction, which are expected to clear spontaneously with simple reassurance. In addition, the drug can cause nausea, dizziness, and faintness associated with a drop in blood pressure, and, theoretically, could change the red blood cell pigment hemoglobin to methemoglobin with a resulting inpairment in the oxygen carrying capacity of the blood.

REFERENCES

1. Ludwig, A. M., Levine, J., & Stark, L. H. *LSD and Alcoholism. A Clinical Study.* Springfield, Ill.: Charles C Thomas, 1970, pp. 13–28, 40–98, 233–244.
2. Dorrance, D. L., Janiger, O., & Teplitz, R. L. Effect of peyote on human chromosomes. Cytogenetic study of the Huichol Indians of Northern Mexico. *Journal of American Medical Association.* 234(3):299–302, 1975.
3. Dobkin de Rios, M. Man, culture and hallucinogens: An overview. In V. Rubin (Ed.), *Cannabis and Culture.* The Hague: Mouton, 1975.
4. Hofmann, F. G., & Hofmann, A. D. *A Handbook on Drug and Alcohol Abuse.* New York: Oxford University Press, 1975, pp. 152–174.
5. Vogel, W. H., & Evans, B. D. Minireview. Structure–activity–relationships of certain hallucinogenic substances based on brain levels. *Life Sciences.* 20:1629–1636, 1977.
6. Jaffe, J. H. Drug addiction and drug abuse. In L. S. Goodman & A. Gilman (Eds.), *The Pharmacological Basis of Therapeutics.* New York: Macmillan, 1975, pp. 284–324.
7. Solursh, L. P. Emergency treatment of acute adverse reactions to hallucinogenic drugs. In P. G. Bourne (Ed.), *A Treatment Manual for Acute Drug Abuse Emergencies.* Washington, D.C.: U.S. Government Printing Office, 1974, pp. 77–79.
8. Medical Letter. Diagnosis and management of reactions to drug abuse. *19*(3):13–16, 1977.
9. Ungerleider, J. T., & Frank, I. M. Emergency treatment of adverse reactions to hallucinogenic drugs. In P. G. Bourne (Ed.), *A Treatment Manual for Acute Drug Abuse Emergencies.* Washington, D.C.: U.S. Government Printing Office, 1974, pp. 73–76.
10. Carino, M. A., & Horita, A. Rapid development of tolerance upon central injection of LSD. *Life Sciences.* 20:49–56, 1977.

11. Cohen, S. (Ed.). Pharmacology of drugs of abuse. *Drug Abuse and Alcoholism Newsletter.* 5(6):1–4, 1976.
12. Brown, J. K., & Malone, M. H. Some U.S. street drug identification programs. *Journal of American Pharmaceutical Association. NS13*(12):670–675, 1973.
13. Bowers, M. B., Jr. Psychoses precipitated by psychotomimetic drugs. A follow-up study. *Archives of General Psychiatry. 34*:832–835, 1977.
14. Blackford, L. *Student Drug Surveys—San Mateo County, California, 1968–1975.* San Mateo County Dept. of Public Health and Welfare, 225-37th Ave., San Mateo, Calif. 94403, 1975.
15. Shapira, J., & Cherubin, C. E. *Drug Abuse: A Guide for the Clinician.* New York: American Elsevier, 1975, p. 368.
16. Taylor, R. L., Maurer, J. I., & Tinklenberg, J. R. Management of "bad trips" in an evolving drug scene. *Journal of the American Medical Association. 213*(3):422–425, 1970.
17. Frosch, W. A., Robbins, E. S., & Stern, M. Untoward reactions to lysergic acid diethylamide (LSD) resulting in hospitalization. *New England Journal of Medicine. 273*(23):1235–1239, 1965.
18. Levy, R. M. Diazepam for LSD intoxication. *Lancet I:*1297, 1971.
19. Woodruff, R. A., Jr., Goodwin, D. W., & Guze, S. B. *Psychiatric Diagnosis.* New York: Oxford University Press, 1974.
20. Cohen, S. (Ed.). Flashbacks. *Drug Abuse and Alcoholism Newsletter. 6*(9):1–3, 1977.
21. Forrest, J. A. H., & Tarala, R. A. 60 hospital admissions due to reactions to lysergide (LSD). *Lancet. II:*1310–1313, 1973.
22. Abruzzi, W. Drug-induced psychosis. *International Journal of the Addictions. 12*(1):183–193, 1977.
23. Shoichet, R. Emergency treatment of acute adverse reactions to hallucinogenic drugs. In P. G. Bourne (Ed.), *A Treatment Manual for Acute Drug Abuse Emergencies.* Washington, D.C.: U.S. Government Printing Office, 1974, pp. 80–82.
24. Friedman, S. A., & Hirsh, S. E. Extreme hyperthermia after LSD ingestion. *Journal of the American Medical Assocation. 217*(11):1549–1550, 1971.
25. Liskow, B. LSD and prolonged psychotic reactions. *American Journal of Psychiatry. 128*(9):1154, 1972.
26. Glass, G. S., & Bowers, M. B. Chronic psychosis associated with long-term psychotomimetic drug abuse. *Archives of General Psychiatry. 23*:97–102, 1970.
27. Ungerleider, J. T. LSD and the courts. *American Journal of Psychiatry. 126*(8):1179, 1970.
28. Grant, I., Mohns, L., Miller, M., & Reitan, R. M. A neuropsychological study of polydrug users. *Archives of General Psychiatry. 33*:973–978, 1976.
29. Robinson, J. T., Chitham, R. G., Greenwood, R. M., & Taylor, J. W. Chromosomal aberrations and LSD. A controlled study in 50 psychiatric patients. *British Journal of Psychiatry. 125*:238–244, 1974.
30. Culver, C. M., & King, F. W. Neuropsychological assessment of undergraduate marihuana and LSD users. *Archives of General Psychiatry. 31*:707–711, 1974.
31. Eller, J. L., & Morton, J. M. Bizarre deformities in offspring of user of lysergic acid diethylamide. *New England Journal of Medicine. 283*(8):395–397, 1970.
32. Emanuel, I., & Ansell, J. S. LSD, intrauterine amputations, and amniotic-band syndrome. *Lancet. July 17:*158–159, 1971.
33. Bloom, A. D. Peyote (mescaline) and human chromosomes. *Journal of the American Medical Association. 234*(3):313, 1975.

34. Bozzetti, L., Jr., Goldsmith, S., & Ungerleider, J. T. The great banana peel hoax. *American Journal of Psychiatry.* 124(5):132–133, 1967.

35. Cohen, S. (Ed.). Angel dust: The pervasive psychedelic. *Drug Abuse and Alcoholism Newsletter.* 5(7):1–3, 1976.

36. Gelenberg, A. J. Psychopharmacology update. *McLean Hospital Journal.* 2(2):89–96, 1977.

37. Schuckit, M. A., & Morrissey, E. R. Propoxyphene and phencyclidine (PCP) use in adolescents. *Journal of Clinical Psychiatry.* 39(1):7–13, 1978.

38. Showalter, C. V., & Thornton, W. E. Clinical pharmacology of phencyclidine toxicity. *American Journal of Psychiatry.* 134:1234–1238, 1977.

39. Cohen, S. (Ed.). PCP. New trends in treatment. *Drug Abuse and Alcoholism Newsletter.* 5(6):1–4, 1978.

40. Yesavage, J. A., & Freman, A. M. Acute PCP intoxication. *Journal of Clinical Psychiatry.* 39:664–666, 1978.

41. Slavney, P R., Rich, G. B., Pearlson, G. D., & McHugh, P. R. Phencyclidine abuse and symptomatic mania. *Biological Psychiatry.* 12:697–700, 1977.

42. Dietz, W. H., Jr., & Stuart, M. J. Nutmeg and prostaglandins. *New England Journal of Medicine.* 294:(9):503, 1976.

43. Schulze, R. G. Nutmeg as a hallucinogen. *New England Journal of Medicine.* 295:174, 1976.

44. Faguet, R. A., Rowland, K. F. "Spice cabinet" intoxication. *American Journal of Psychiatry.* 135:860–861, 1973.

45. Fink, P. J., Goldman, M. J., & Lyons, I. Morning glory seed psychosis. *Archives of General Psychiatry.* 15:209–213, 1966.

46. Domino, E. F. The hallucinogens. In R. W. Richter (Ed.), *Medical Aspects of Drug Abuse.* New York: Harper & Row, 1975, p. 4.

47. Block, S. H. The grocery store high. *American Journal of Psychiatry.* 135(1):126, 1978.

48. Brodsky, L., & Zuniga, J. Nitrous oxide: A psychotogenic agent. *Comprehensive Psychiatry.* 16(2):185–188, 1975.

49. Nickerson, M. Vasodilator drugs. In L. S. Goodman & A. Gilman (Eds.), *The Pharmacological Basis of Therapeutics.* New York: Macmillan, 1965, pp. 734–738.

50. Cohen, S. (Ed.). Amyl nitrite rediscovered. *Drug Abuse and Alcoholism Newsletter.* 7(1):1–3, 1978.

Glues, Solvents, and Aerosols

9.1. INTRODUCTION

9.1.1. General Comments

This short chapter deals with a heterogeneous group of industrial substances[1] that share the ability to produce generalized CNS depression.[2] While intermittent use of solvents was noted in the last century,[2] more widespread misuse began with inhalation of model airplane glue in the early 1960s.[3] Despite efforts of the hobby industry to modify their products by removing some of the more toxic substances and adding an irritating smell, abuses have continued, and intoxication through inhalation has spread to aerosol propellants and industrial solvents.[2]

The more frequently abused agents and their contents, presented in Table 9.1, include cleaning solvents such as carbon tetrachloride, toluene, gasoline, lighter fluids, nail polish, and the fluorinated hydrocarbons used in aerosols. These products are popular because they induce euphoria and are readily available, cheap, legal, and easy to conceal. The

Table 9.1
Some Commonly Used Agents[1,2,12]

Glues	Toluene, naphtha, acetates, hexane, benzene, xylene, chloroform, etc.
Cleaning solutions	Trichloroethylene, petroleum products, carbon tetrachloride
Nail polish removers	Acetone, etc.
Lighter fluids	Naphtha, aliphatic hydrocarbons, etc.
Paints and paint thinners	Toluene, butylacetate, acetone, naphtha, methanol, ethanol, etc.
Aerosols	Fluorinated hydrocarbons, nitrous oxide, etc.
Other petroleum products	Gasoline, benzene, toluene, petroleum ether

onset of mental change occurs rapidly and disappears fairly quickly, and, with the exception of headache, serious hangovers are usually not seen.[4]

9.1.2. Pharmacology

9.1.2.1. General Characteristics

The solvents are all fat-soluble organic substances that easily pass through the blood–brain barrier to produce a change in the state of consciousness similar to more mild Stage I or II levels of anesthesia.[1] It is difficult to make detailed generalizations, as the substances themselves are diverse in structure, and most commercial products contain a combination of solvents along with other chemicals[5]; however, metabolism usually occurs in both the kidneys and the liver.

9.1.2.2. Predominant Effects

The usual "high" begins within minutes and lasts a quarter to three-quarters of an hour, during which the individual feels giddy and light-headed.[2] Most users relate a decrease in inhibitions along with a floating sensation, misperceptions or illusions, clouding of thoughts and drowsiness, and occasionally amnesia during the height of the inhalation episode.[1–3]

Acute intoxication is accompanied by a variety of potentially disturbing physiological symptoms as noted in Table 9.2, including irritation of the eyes, sensitivity to light, double vision, ringing in the ears, irritation of the lining or mucous membranes of the nose and mouth, and a

Table 9.2
Common Signs and Symptoms of Acute Intoxication[1,2,12]

Sensory	Light sensitivity
	Eye irritation
	Double vision
	Ringing ears
Respiratory	Sneezing
	Runny nose
	Cough
Gastrointestinal	Nausea
	Vomiting
	Diarrhea
	Loss of appetite
Other	Chest pain
	Abnormal heart rhythm
	Muscle and joint aches

cough.[6,7] The abuser may also complain of nausea, vomiting, and diarrhea and become faint or (especially with a fluorinated hydrocarbon aerosol) may demonstrate cardiac beating irregularities or arrhythmias.[2,8] Intoxication is usually associated with a slowing of the brain waves on electroencephalogram to an 8–10/second pattern.[1]

9.1.2.3. Tolerance and Dependence

Toleration of higher doses of solvents appears to develop fairly quickly, but there is little evidence of cross-tolerance between substances.[2] Withdrawal symptoms do not develop, even with protracted use.[1,2]

9.1.3. Epidemiology and Patterns of Abuse

Solvents are usually taken intermittently,[4] with the highest prevalence among adolescent boys involved in other delinquent acts.[1,2,9] The teenagers tend to abandon use of solvents as they mature or to move on to other substances, but a small percentage continues with these as their drugs of choice.[1,10] Although the actual scope of use of the solvents is unknown, a survey done in the 1970s indicated that as many as 20% of adolescent girls and as high as one-third of adolescent boys in an urban setting have used solvents at least once, with the percentage of continuing users *decreasing* from junior high school to high school and into college.[11]

Solvents are usually taken by groups of young people, using any one of a variety of modes of administration. For the glues, it is common to inhale from a paper or plastic bag, perhaps increasing the intensity of the fumes by gentle warming. Unfortunately, this also markedly increases the chances of suffocation, especially when plastic bags are used.[1,2] Liquids, such as the industrial solvents and paint thinners, can be inhaled directly from a container or by sniffing a cloth or placing the cloth in the mouth, while gasoline is sometimes inhaled directly from gas tanks.[1,2,4] Propellants may be inhaled directly, but most users attempt to separate out particulate contents by straining the gases through a cloth.[2,4] In the survey alluded to above, three-quarters of users reported inhaling a substance from a plastic bag, and over half used paint, 40% glue, 37% gasoline, 27% nail polish, and 25% lacquer.[11]

9.2. EMERGENCY PROBLEMS

The most common emergency situations seen with the solvents are toxic reactions, organic brain syndromes, and medical complications.

9.2.1. Panic Reactions (See Section 1.5.1.)

Because the period of intoxication is short (15–45 minutes), panic states usually abate by the time an individual would seek professional care.

9.2.2. Flashbacks (See Section 1.5.2.)

With the exception of possible residual organic brain syndromes, flashbacks are not known to occur with these drugs.

9.2.3. Toxic Reactions (See Section 12.4.)

9.2.3.1. The Clinical Picture

9.2.3.1.1. History

The patient usually experiences the very abrupt (within minutes) onset of severe physical distress while inhaling a solvent. This is usually done as part of a group activity involving young teenagers.

9.2.3.1.2. Physical Signs and Symptoms

A life-threatening toxic picture characterized by respiratory depression and cardiac arrhythmias can follow the administration of solvents. The result may be a rapid loss of consciousness and sudden death.[12] There is also a chance of death from suffocation in those individuals who inhale deeply from a plastic bag, which then collapses.[2]

9.2.3.1.3. Psychological State

The physically ill individual may present with anxiety and some level of mental impairment ranging from OBS to coma.

9.2.3.1.4. Relevant Laboratory Tests

These are rarely helpful in establishing the diagnosis. It is important, however, to carry out a thorough physical examination and to establish baseline vital signs. It is also necessary to monitor cardiac functioning through an EKG and to establish red and white blood cell counts (see Table 1.5), as well as the level of liver function and kidney function (see Section 9.2.7.).

9.2.3.2. Treatment

There are no specific antidotes for the solvent overdose. Treatment consists of offering good supportive care, symptomatically controlling arrhythmias, and aiding the respirations. Thus, therapy would be similar to the general life supports outlined for opiates in Section 6.2.3., except that naloxone (Narcan) has no use here.

9.2.4. Psychosis

Any change in mentation occurring with the solvents is likely to involve an organic brain syndrome, not the delusions and/or hallucinations that might be seen with stimulants or depressants. One possible exception is the occasional violent outburst during intoxication from solvents that may be analogous to alcohol-related pathological intoxication[4] (see Section 4.2.4.). Treatment is aimed at controlling behavior for the short period of intoxication through reassurance and physical or pharmacologic controls, such as diazepam (Valium) 15–30 mg or more by mouth, or chlordiazepoxide 25–50 mg or more which can be repeated in one hour, if needed.

9.2.5. Organic Brain Syndrome

9.2.5.1. The Clinical Picture (See Section 1.5.5.)

Frequently, individuals abusing solvents present with a rapid onset of confusion and disorientation. The patient may have a rash around the nose or mouth from inhaling, may have the odor of a solvent on his breath, and may have been found in a semiconscious state with solvents near him or be brought in by somebody who knows that he has been taking solvents.

9.2.5.2. Treatment

This is usually a short-lived organic brain syndrome clearing within a matter of hours. As in any delirium state, treatment centers around reassurance, elimination of any ambiguous or misleading stimuli, such as shadows or whispers, protecting the patient from the consequences of hostile outbursts, and providing a generally supportive environment.

9.2.6. Withdrawal

No clinically relevant withdrawal syndrome from solvents has been described.

9.2.7. Medical Problems

9.2.7.1. Clinical Pictures

These substances interfere with the normal functioning of most body systems. However, because abuse is generally intermittent and relatively short-lived and the typical user is young and healthy, permanent sequelae are relatively rare. Nonetheless, the range of problems must be noted, as deaths do occur. The medical disorders associated with the solvents include the following:

1. Cardiac irregularities or arrhythmias can be seen with acute inhalation, especially with aerosol use.[8]

2. Hepatitis with possible liver failure has been noted following chronic exposure to solvents.[2,12,13]

3. Kidney failure may be seen with chronic abuse of toluene and benzene.[2,6,13]

4. Transient impairment in tests of lung functioning may be noted immediately after inhalation.[14]

5. Decreased production of all types of blood cells may occur and may result in a life-threatening aplastic anemia.[6,13]

6. Skeletal muscle weakness may develop as a result of muscle destruction, especially with toluene abuse.[6]

7. Transient mild stomach or gastrointestinal upsets can be seen with any of these substances.[6]

8. Peripheral neuropathies have been reported, especially a lead-induced nerve damage to the hands and feet associated with chronic inhalation of gasoline.

9. There is *anecdotal* evidence that these substances produce permanent CNS damage,[2,4] but reports in the literature are not consistent.[1]

9.2.7.2. Treatment

Most of these disorders are transient and disappear with general supportive care. In the case of severe liver or kidney damage, treatment consists of that used for insults to these organs from any source. Any patient presenting with an encephalopathy should be carefully evaluated for other causes of the OBS, including intracranial bleeding.

REFERENCES

1. Glaser, F. B. Inhalation psychosis and related states. In P. G. Bourne (Ed.), *A Treatment Manual for Acute Drug Abuse Emergencies*. Washington, D.C.: U.S. Government Printing Office, 1974, pp. 95–104.

2. Hoffman, F. G. *A Handbook on Drug and Alcohol Abuse.* New York: Oxford University Press, 1975.
3. Glatt, M. M. Abuse of solvents "for kicks." *The Lancet I:*485, Feb. 1977.
4. Cohen, S. Glue sniffing. *Journal of the American Medical Association. 231*(6):653–654, 1975.
5. Cohen, S. Inhalant abuse. *Drug Abuse and Alcoholism Newsletter. 6*(9). San Diego: The Vista Hill Foundation, 1975.
6. Keeler, M. H., & Reifler, C. B. The occurrence of glue sniffing on a university campus. *College Health. 16:*69–70, 1967.
7. Lewis, P. W., & Patterson, D. Acute and chronic effects of the voluntary inhalation of certain commercial volatile solvents by juveniles. *Journal of Drug Issues.* 162–175, 1974.
8. Jaffe, J. H. Drug addiction and drug abuse. In L. S. Goodman & A. Gilman (Eds.), *The Pharmacological Basis of Therapeutics.* New York: Macmillan, 1975, pp. 284–324.
9. Watson, J. M. "Glue-sniffing" in profile. *The Practitioner. 218:*255–259, 1977.
10. Faillace, L. A., & Guynn, R. W. Abuse of organic solvents. *Psychosomatics. 17*(4): 188–189, 1976.
11. Albeson, H., Cohen, R., Schrayer, D., *et al.* Drug experience, attitudes, and related behavior among adolescents and adults. In The National Commission on Marijuana and Drug Abuse (Ed.), *The Technical Papers of the Second Report of the National Commission on Marijuana and Drug Abuse,* Vol 1. Washington, D.C.: U.S. Government Printing Office, 1972.
12. Adriani, J. Drug dependence in hospitalized patients. In P. G. Bourne (Ed.), *A Treatment Manual for Acute Drug Abuse Emergencies.* Washington, D.C.: U.S. Government Printing Office, 1974, pp. 125–136.
13. Stybel, L. J. Deliberate hydrocarbon inhalation among low socioeconomic adolescents not necessarily apprehended by the police. *The International Journal of the Addictions. 11*(2):345–361, 1976.
14. Fagan, D. G., & Forrest, J. B. "Sudden sniffing death" after inhalation of domestic lipid-aerosol. *The Lancet II:*361, 1977.

CHAPTER 10

Over-the-Counter (O/C) Drugs

10.1. INTRODUCTION

10.1.1. General Comments

The over-the-counter (O/C) drugs discussed in this chapter include non-prescription hypnotics (containing atropinelike [anticholinergic] substances and antihistamines), nonprescription antianxiety drugs (usually containing substances similar to the O/C hypnotics), O/C analgesics (containing aspirin, phenacetin, and aspirinlike products), nonprescription stimulants and diet pills, and most laxatives. Because of the wide array of substances involved, each subsection represents a minichapter following the usual chapter format.

The history of O/C medications is a long one, as controls on drug availability are relatively recent and, at the turn of the century, anyone could purchase opium, cocaine, and other potent substances without a prescription.[1,2] Currently, there are many nonprescription drugs that have been poorly evaluated and subsequently are of questionable efficacy. On the other hand, most are capable of producing physical and emotional pathology when taken either in excessive doses or in combination with other medications or alcohol.

Unfortunately, health care practitioners and the general public have limited knowledge of the dangers of these substances. Most people receive their information from advertisements or pharmacists, rather than from physicians.[3] The result is the very heavy use, and frequent misuse, of these drugs, with resulting pathology coming to light in both emergency and general practice settings. Because of these common problems and the large variety of substances involved, the reader is encouraged to review other discussions of the O/C drugs.[4,5]

138

10.1.2. Epidemiology and Pattern of Abuse

There are more than 500,000 different O/C preparations.[3] At least 28% of the adult population of the United States use these substances (not including aspirin), 12% taking caffeinated stimulants, 11% sleep medications, and 5% antianxiety drugs.[6] Many users combine O/C products with prescription drugs and alcohol.

Over-the-counter substances are used by all elements of society and must be considered a part of the differential diagnosis of emergency room problems in any patient; however, the most frequent user tends to be the white, middle-class woman.[1] Use of O/C substances is noted in 7–10% of emergency room cases, two-thirds of these involving analgesics, and 17% sedatives.[1,2] The O/C drugs accounted for approximately 2% of the accidental overdose deaths and almost 3% of the suicides in one locale.[2]

10.2. ATROPINELIKE (ANTICHOLINERGIC)/ANTIHISTAMINIC DRUGS (SEDATIVES/HYPNOTICS)

10.2.1. General Comments

The atropine-type drugs have long been used in medicine as aids in anesthesia (blocking some of the effects of anesthetic agents on the heart) and in treatment for a variety of digestive upsets, heart problems, and eye diseases. They are also used in the treatment of motion sickness, Parkinson's disease, urinary problems, and the symptoms of the common cold.[7] The atropinic substances, because of their side effect of lethargy, are found in the O/C hypnotics and daytime sedatives (usually in the form of scopolamine) in doses ranging from 0.125 mg to 0.5 mg. At these levels, controlled studies have not shown these drugs to be effective sleep aids. Furthermore, doses as low as 10 mg of scopolamine can be fatal, especially in children.[5]

Only two of the more commonly purchased sleep aids (Sleep-Eze and Sominex) contain scopolamine (as shown in Table 10.1), but all contain antihistamines. These latter drugs work primarily to inhibit release of histamines during allergic reactions, but drowsiness occurs as a side effect. However, while most of the O/C sleep aids contain between 15 and 50 mg of the antihistamine methapyrilene, 50-mg doses are probably no better than a placebo in producing sleep.

As was true with the sleep aids, controlled studies indicate that O/C sedatives (such as Compoz) are no more effective than placebo or aspirin, and they are significantly less effective than chlordiazepoxide (Librium). However, compared to aspirin and placebo, patients taking Compoz have increased rates of side effects, including sleepiness, dizziness, dry mouth, nausea, and confusion.

Table 10.1
Some Commonly Used O/C Hypnotics and
Antianxiety Drugs

Trade name	Contents
Hypnotics	
Sominex	Scopolamine: 0.25 mg/tablet and 0.5 mg/capsule
	Antihistamine: 25/mg tablet and 50 mg/capsule
	Analgesic: salicylamide, 200 mg
Sleep-Eze	Scopolamine: 0.125 mg
	Antihistamine: 25 mg
Nytol	Antihistamine: 25 mg/tablet and 50 mg/capsule
	Analgesic: salicylamide, 200 mg/tablet, 380 mg/capsule
Sedacaps	Antihistamine: 25 mg
Sleepinal	Antihistamine: 50 mg
Antianxiety	
Compoz	Antihistamine: 25 mg
Nervine	Antihistamine: 25 mg

10.2.2. Pharmacology

The antihistamines and the anticholinergic drugs, atropine or scopolamine, are rapidly absorbed when taken orally and have a rapid onset of action.[7] The anticholinergic drugs work by attenuating the effects of the transmitter substance, acetylcholine. This makes them useful in treating overdoses of certain muscarinic mushrooms, hence leading to the additional label of *antimuscarinic agents*.[7] Atropine is found in a variety of plants, including deadly nightshade, jimson weed, loco weed, stinkweed, and angel's trumpet, while scopolamine occurs naturally in the henbane shrub.[7-9] These substances are very potent, with doses as low as 1 mg producing clinical effects, including an increased heart rate, blurred vision (from paralysis of the muscles that control the lens of the eye), headache, dry mouth, hot skin, and some clouding of levels of consciousness.

The antihistamines, as the name implies, work by antagonizing the actions of histamine released by the body during allergic reactions.

10.2.3. Epidemiology

It has been estimated that 18 million Americans have used O/C hypnotics or sedatives, with at least 4 million having taken one of the substances in the prior six months. The rate of administration of these substances is higher in women, with two-thirds of users being over age 35 and 50% over age 50.[2] For the O/C tranquilizers, the average user tends to be younger, usually under age 35.

10.2.4. Emergency Situations

Emergencies usually result from inadvertent overdose, deliberate misuse of the drugs in an attempt to achieve hallucinations, or multiple-drug interactions. Therefore, the most frequently noted syndromes in the emergency room are toxic reactions, psychoses, and organic brain syndromes. In addition, there are common, usually reversible, medical problems. It is important to note that many prescription drugs with anticholinergic properties (for example benztropine [Cogentin]) might also be abused and produce similar psychoses or organic brain syndromes.

10.2.4.1. Panic Reactions (See Section 1.6.1.)

10.2.4.1.1. Clinical Picture

A panic occurring at normal drug doses is unlikely, although a patient might present with complaints of muddled thinking related to these drugs.

10.2.4.1.2. Treatment

Reassurance should be enough to allay the patient's fears and decrease the level of discomfort.

10.2.4.2. Toxic Reactions (See Sections 1.6.2., 2.2.3., 6.2.3., and 12.4.)

10.2.4.2.1. Clinical Picture

The toxic reaction for the O/C antianxiety and hypnotic drugs, as well as for benztropine (Cogentin) is usually time-limited, disappearing in 2–48 hours. The clinical picture can be confusing and life-threatening, especially if multiple substances have been taken or if the drug involved is a hallucinogen.[9]

1. *History.* The onset of symptoms varies from a few minutes, as seen in an overdose, to the more gradual evolution of signs of confusion and physical pathology in an elderly patient consuming close to the "normal" doses of an O/C sedative. The patient is rarely a member of the "street culture."

2. *Physical signs and symptoms.* Agitation and anxiety may be accompanied by a very rapid heart rate and other anticholinergic signs, such as dry mouth, difficulty swallowing, abdominal distension, urinary reten-

tion, blurred vision and sensitivity to light, and a rash covering the face and upper neck. There may also be an elevation of blood pressure.

3. *Psychological state.* The patient usually presents in a state of agitation and may evidence varying degrees of an OBS.

4. *Relevant laboratory tests.* The signs of confusion along with the stigmata of an anticholinergic crisis (e.g., dry mouth, warm dry skin, etc.) usually establish the diagnosis. However, a toxicologic screen (10 ml of blood or 50 ml of urine) may be useful. As with any patient with unstable vital signs and a level of organic impairment, it is necessary to establish baseline levels of functioning and to rule out other physical causes, such as infections, trauma, tumors, etc.

10.2.4.2.2. Treatment

Therapy for the toxic reaction involves general support, symptomatic treatment of physiological reactions, such as the elevated body temperature, and a direct attack on the anticholinergic syndrome. The factors to consider are listed below but their order of importance may change with specific clinical situations.

1. Attention must be paid to maintenance of an adequate airway, adequate circulation, and the control of any traumatic lesions or bleeding. This treatment is described in greater depth in Sections 2.2.3., and 6.2.3.

2. A rapid physical exam and careful monitoring of vital signs must be carried out.

3. Because these drugs are usually taken orally, saline gastric lavage might be beneficial, continuing the procedure until a clear return from the stomach is noted. However, if the patient is comatose or semi-comatose, lavage may be done safely only with an inflated cuff on a tracheal tube.

4. Relatively normal body temperature must be maintained by using a hypothermic blanket or alcohol/ice soaks, if necessary.[7,9]

5. The anticholinergic syndrome is best treated directly by the antidote physostigmine, given by slow IV injection of 1–4 mg (0.5–1.0mg/kg for children).[7] The dose can be repeated in 15 minutes if the patient does not respond; and once improvement is noted, it may be repeated every 1–3 hours until symptoms abate.[7,10] With this regimen, one can expect improvement in the mental status and the physiological symptoms, although there is no reversal in pupillary dilatation until the anticholinergic drugs wear off.

6. It is wise to avoid all other drugs, if possible. However, if the patient is exceptionally excitable, one might use diazepam (Valium) in doses of 5–20 mg given orally or IM, or chlordiazepoxide (Librium) in doses of 10–25 mg orally. The dose may be repeated in an hour, if necessary.

7. It is imperative that you avoid giving drugs that themselves have anticholinergic side effects. This rules out all of the antipsychotic drugs, such as chlorpromazine (Thorazine).[7,9]

8. No specific treatment is known for the CNS depression resulting from the antihistaminic portion of the overdose, and care is symptomatic.

10.2.4.3. Psychoses (See Section 1.6.4.)

10.2.4.3.1. Clinical Picture

Although this topic is discussed separately for ease of reference, the psychosis here is simply an intense toxic reaction. It consists of hallucinations, frequently visual, along with illusions (misinterpretation of normal sensory stimuli) and is usually accompanied by confusion.[9]

10.2.4.3.2. Treatment

The treatment and prognosis are the same as outlined above in Section 10.2.4.2.2.

10.2.4.4. Organic Brain Syndrome (See Section 1.5.5.)

A patient presenting with confusion and the physical signs of an anticholinergic syndrome (e.g., dry mouth, dilated pupils, rapid heart rate, warm skin) could be labeled as a toxic reaction. The entire clinical picture, course, and treatment are identical to those outlined in Section 10.2.4.2.

10.2.4.5. Medical Problems

10.2.4.5.1. Clinical Picture

These also reflect a toxic anticholinergic syndrome. One can expect an inability to pass urine (due to a flaccid bladder), abdominal distension secondary to a halting of peristalsis, blurred vision, and dry skin and mucous membranes.

10.2.4.5.2. Treatment

The treatment is symptomatic and is achieved by general supportive care and use of physostigmine as described in Section 10.2.4.2.2.

10.3. COLD AND ALLERGY PRODUCTS

These substances contain antihistamines, analgesics, decongestants, expectorants, cough suppressants, and anticholinergic substances. The major clinical syndromes are similar to those seen for the atropinelike drugs. Treatment is usually symptomatic or, if anticholinergic drugs are involved, through the use of physostigmine (Section 10.2.4.2.2.).[11]

In addition, CNS depression, especially respiratory impairment, may follow the excessive doses of cough suppressants. In that instance, one can expect to see a mild form of some of the syndromes noted for the opiates (See Section 6.2.3.).

10.4. BROMIDES

10.4.1. General Comments

This element has been in use since approximately 1860, when it was one of the only anticonvulsant and antianxiety drugs available.[12] Problems of misuse have been noted since the 1920s, and in the 1940s and 1950s bromide intoxication was felt to be a major precipitant of psychiatric hospitalization.[13] Until recent years, a variety of substances used as sedatives contained bromides, including Miles Nervine, Bromo Seltzer, and other O/C hypnotics or sedatives.

10.4.2. Pharmacology

With chronic bromide use, psychopathology is likely to develop slowly, reflecting a half-life of approximately 12 days. If an individual were to take 16.5 mEq of bromide a day (the maximal amount allowable in O/C medications), he could be expected to develop intoxication in eight days, or sooner in children or patients with renal problems.

10.4.3. Emergency Problems

While bromides have not been proved to be effective O/C sleep aids, they were, *until recent years*, widely available. They are no longer on the market.

10.4.3.1. Toxic Reactions (See Section 12.4.)

10.4.3.1.1. Clinical Picture

1. *History.* The usual patient with bromide intoxication presents with the very gradual onset (over days, weeks, or months) of both physical and psychological impairment resulting from chronic ingestion of O/C preparations containing bromide. Even with the phasing out of bromides in medications, cases still persist from ingestion of drugs stored in the medicine cabinet or from contaminated water.[14]

2. *Physical signs and symptoms.* These are usually mild and consist of a

fine tremor, a macular–papular skin rash, along with *neurological problems* such as slurred speech, impaired coordination, and dizziness.

3. *Psychological state.* Toxic disturbances include any of a wide variety of emotional problems. These range from irritability to all grades of confusion (culminating in an organic brain syndrome), to any level of depression, and even maniclike behavior (hyperactivity and inability to organize thoughts.)

4. *Relevant laboratory tests.* As with all organicities, especially in the elderly, it is necessary to rule out physical abnormalities through the proper blood chemistries and counts (see Table 1.5) and through an adequate physical and neurological examination, as well as evaluation of CNS and cardiac functioning. A bromide level over 10–20 mEq/l indicates probable toxicity with definite impairment noted at 80 mEq/l.

10.4.3.1.2. Treatment

Treatment consists of general supportive care and the IV administration of either sodium or ammonium chloride, or possibly normal saline, in doses of 330 ml per hour, for 2 liters, which, for younger healthy individuals, is then alternated with 5% dextrose in saline.[15]

10.5. O/C ANALGESICS

10.5.1. General Comments

These substances usually contain aspirin, aspirinlike substances (such as phenacetin, acetaminophen), and caffeine. They are used for relief from minor pains, such as headache, and—for aspirin and aspirin compounds—for the treatment of some chronic inflammatory disorders such as arthritis. Abuse reflects psychological dependence, as these drugs are not physically addicting and do not produce hallucinations or changes in the level of consciousness.

10.5.2. Pharmacology

Aspirin is both an analgesic and an antiinflammatory substance that is readily absorbed orally, while phenacetin and acetaminophen are analgesic but not antiinflammatory. Caffeine is discussed below under the O/C stimulants in Section 10.7. Some of the analgesics also contain antiacidic compounds such as sodium bicarbonate (e.g., Bromo Seltzer and Vanquish).

10.5.3. Epidemiology and Pattern of Misuse

Analgesic use has doubled in the last 10 years,[15] with a resulting 33 million users in the United States, 20 million of whom take the drug each month. In one survey of almost 3,000 individuals, 15% of the women and 18% of the men ingested aspirin daily, [16,17] with the rate of administration exhibiting no marked age or sex pattern. In a survey of drug-involved emergency room visits, 64% of those with a major problem with analgesics were taking aspirin, and 46% of those drug-involved emergencies were suicide attempts. There are now more than 300 products containing aspirin in the O/C market.[2]

10.5.4. Emergency Situations

The major emergency problems for analgesic users are toxic overdoses and medical disorders resulting from chronic use. Older individuals are especially liable to misuse analgesics and are at high risk for adverse reactions.[18]

10.5.4.1. Panic Reactions

These are virtually nonexistent with these drugs.

10.5.4.2. Flashbacks

These are not noted with the analgesics.

10.5.4.3. Toxic Reactions (See Section 1.6.3.)

10.5.4.3.1. Clinical Picture

Overdosage with O/C analgesics usually results in a profound acid–base imbalance, ringing in the ears, and electrolyte problems. This problem is most often seen in adolescents engaging in a deliberate overdose, usually in a spur-of-the-moment reaction to a life situation.

10.5.4.3.2. Treatment

The picture tends to be relatively benign, responding to general supportive measures. Diuresis (Section 2.2.3.2.) is rarely needed. However, as in any emergency situation, unforeseen complications, such as hospital-acquired infections or kidney failure, can occur and may be fatal.

10.5.4.4. Psychoses

Psychoses are rarely, if ever, seen with these drugs.

10.5.4.5. Organic Brain Syndrome (See Section 1.5.5.)

An OBS occurring with O/C analgesics is usually the result of acid–base or electrolyte imbalance. It is temporary and will clear with supportive care.

10.5.4.6. Medical Complications

10.5.4.6.1. Clinical Picture

The medical problems seen with analgesics vary from acute, usually benign, reactions, to more permanent responses due to chronic drug misuse. Acutely, aspirin may cause gastrointestinal upset, bleeding, gastric ulcers, minor changes in blood coagulability, asthmatic attacks, and skin reactions.[2]

Chronic use of O/C analgesics can be associated with anemia, peptic ulcers, upper gastrointestinal bleeding, and renal disease. Phenacetin, in chronic high doses, can produce kidney failure and chronic anemia.

10.5.4.6.2. Treatment

Treatment is symptomatic and supportive, based on the individual clinical picture.

10.6. LAXATIVE ABUSE

10.6.1. General Comments

Laxatives consist of a wide variety of substances that act through diverse methods, including increasing bulk in the colon and increasing colon motility. They can be generally subdivided into salines, bulk producers, emolients, lubricants (e.g., mineral oil), and hyperosmotic agents (e.g., glycerin).[19]

10.6.2. Pharmacology

The pharmacology, of course, differs with the specific laxative. Those most likely to cause systemic problems contain phenolphthalein, which, when absorbed, can cause cardiac and respiratory distress in susceptible individuals.

10.6.3. Epidemiology and Pattern of Misuse

Laxative use has become entrenched in Western societies, especially in individuals of advanced age.[18] It has been estimated that more than

30% of people over age 60 take a weekly dose of a cathartic with the goal of achieving daily bowel movements.

10.6.4. Emergency Situations—Medical Disorders

Laxatives are not physically addicting, do not cause changes in level of consciousness, and have no direct effect on the CNS; consequently the major problems are medical.

1. Effects of laxative misuse include diarrhea, abdominal pain, thirst, muscular weakness, cramps secondary to hypokalemia, and the characteristic radiological appearance of a distended and flaccid colon.

2. Mineral oil laxatives may impede the absorption of some minerals and fat-soluble vitamins, producing a hypovitaminosis syndrome.

3. Saline cathartics can also result in dehydration and electrolyte imbalance, with important consequences for individuals with preexisting cardiac disorders.

4. Other disorders that can be seen after chronic overuse of laxatives include melanosis coli, fecal impaction from a flaccid colon, osteomalacia, and protein loss.[19]

10.7. STIMULANTS (See Chapter 5 for prescription stimulants.)

10.7.1. General Comments

These substances, usually containing caffeine as their major active ingredient, are mostly used by people who work unusual hours, such as cross-country truck drivers and students preparing for exams. Similar emergency problems can be seen for the O/C asthma products, especially those containing stramonium.

10.7.2. Pharmacology

Caffeine is a drug whose properties have been recognized for centuries.[2] Found naturally in teas, coffees, colas, and cocoa, caffeine produces mild stimulating effects. With doses in excess of 100 mg (1–2 cups of coffee contain 150–250 mg), people begin to experience a slightly increased thought flow, an enhancement in motor activity, and a decreased drowsiness and fatigue. Accompanying these psychological changes are increases in heart rate and blood pressure, along with GI irritability. Fatal overdosage from caffeine would require 10 g (70–100 cups of coffee).

10.7.3. Epidemiology and Pattern of Misuse

Not counting beverages, 16 million Americans have used O/C stimulants. Two-thirds of the users are male, but all races and socioeconomic groups are represented. There is an increased level of use among students and employed males.

The drugs containing caffeine as their major ingredient are No Doz (which has 100 mg per tablet) and Vivarin (which has 250 mg per tablet). Other drugs are Come Back, Enerjets, Tirend, and Chaser for hangover.[20]

10.7.4. Emergency Situations

The most frequent emergencies include panic reactions and medical problems. There is no evidence that these substances are physiologically addicting, no evidence of flashbacks, and no information to indicate that they produce psychoses. Of course, in high enough doses, they can produce an organic brain syndrome, but this is extremely rare.

10.7.4.1. Panic (See Section 1.6.1. and 5.2.1.)

10.7.4.1.1. Clinical Picture

Stimulants can produce an increased blood pressure, a rapid heart rate, and palpitations, which may be perceived by the individual as a heart attack.

10.7.4.1.2. Treatment

Treatment is exactly the same as that for any panic reaction (Sections 5.2.1., and 7.2.1.):

1. Carry out a rapid physical examination, including an EKG to rule out physical pathology.
2. Draw blood (10 ml) or collect urine (50 cc) for a toxicologic screen.
3. Center treatment on gentle reassurance.

10.7.4.1.3. Medical Problems

The major medical disorders seen with stimulants include exacerbation of preexisting heart disease or hypertension and precipitation of pain in individuals with ulcers. Treatment is symptomatic.

10.8. WEIGHT CONTROL PRODUCTS

10.8.1. General Comments

These substances are of limited, if any, value in weight control. As is true of the prescription CNS stimulants, any weight reduction that occurs tends to be temporary. Most O/C weight control products contain either a relatively weak sympathomimetic-type drug (phenylpropanolamine), a local anesthetic (benzocaine), or a bulk producer (methylcellulose).

10.8.2. Pharmacology

Phenylpropanolamine is a sympathomimetic or adrenalinelike agent similar to amphetamine, which produces an adrenaline-type response along with weak CNS stimulation. In the suggested dosages, it is of questionable efficacy in decreasing appetite. The drug is associated with nervousness, restlessness, insomnia, headaches, palpitations, and increased blood pressure.

Benzocaine is a local anesthetic that is included in some weight control products in an attempt to decrease hunger. There is no evidence that this drug is effective in decreasing appetite.

Methylcellulose produces bulk and thus a feeling of fullness in the stomach. However, this substance is no more effective than a low-calorie, high-residue diet, and it does have a danger of producing esophageal obstruction.

10.8.3. Epidemiology and Pattern of Misuse

There is very little, if any, evidence available on the patterns of misuse of weight control substances. One would estimate the most frequent users to be young to middle-aged women.

10.8.4. Emergency Situations

Although there are few data, it is possible that, in high enough doses, phenylpropanolamine could produce emergency situations similar to those outlined under the CNS stimulants (Section 5.2.).

Methylcellulose can produce esophageal obstruction, especially in individuals who already have esophageal or gastric disease. This should be treated symptomatically.

10.9. GENERAL CONCLUSIONS

Misuse of O/C drugs, whether done deliberately or inadvertently, can result in toxic reactions characterized by panic, OBS, or medical complications. These substances must be considered whenever an individual presents to an emergency room with a fairly rapid evolution of an OBS along with neurological signs. In evaluating all patients, it is important to gather an adequate history of O/C drug preparations, being especially wary regarding older or more debilitated individuals.

REFERENCES

1. Chambers, C. D., Inciardi, J. A., & Siegal, H. A. *Chemical Coping: A Report on Legal Drug Use in the United States.* New York: Spectrum Publications, 1975.

2. Inciardi, J. A. Over-the-counter drugs: Epidemiology, adverse reactions, overdose deaths, and mass media promotion. *Addictive Diseases: An International Journal.* 3(2):253–272, 1977.

3. Boatman, D. W., & Gagnon, J. P. The pharmacist as an information source for nonprescription drugs. *Journal of Drug Issues.* 7(2):183–193, 1977.

4. Inglefinger, F. J. Those "ingredients most used by doctors." *New England Journal of Medicine.* 295:616–617, 1976.

5. Caro, J. P. Sleep aid and sedative products. In APhA Project Staff (Eds.), *Handbook of Nonprescription Drugs,* 5th Ed. Washington, D.C.: American Pharmaceutical Association, 1977.

6. Brecher, E. M. *Licit and Illicit Drugs.* Boston: Little, Brown, 1972.

7. Innes, I. R., & Nickerson, M. Atropine, scopolamine, and related antimuscarinic drugs. In L. S. Goodman & A. Gilman (Eds.), *The Pharmacological Basis of Therapeutics,* 5th Ed. New York: Macmillan, 1975, pp. 495–511.

8. Hall, R. C. W., Popkin, M. K., & McHenry, L. E. Angel's trumpet psychosis: A central nervous system anticholinergic syndrome. *American Journal of Psychiatry.* 134(3):312–314, 1977.

9. Hoffman, F. G. *A Handbook on Drug and Alcohol Abuse.* New York: Oxford University Press, 1975.

10. Ullman, K. C., & Groh, R. H. Identification and treatment of acute psychotic states secondary to the usage of over-the-counter sleeping preparations. *American Journal of Psychiatry.* 128(10):64–68, 1972.

11. Cormier, J. F., & Bryant, B. G. Cold and allergy products. In APhA Project Staff (Eds.), *Handbook of Nonprescription Drugs,* 5th Ed. Washington, D.C.: American Pharmaceutical Association, 1977.

12. Harvey, S. C. Miscellaneous agents. In L. S. Goodman & A. Gilman (Eds.), *The Pharmacological Basis of Therapeutics,* 5th Ed. New York: Macmillan, 1975, pp. 388–391.

13. Burch, E. A., Jr. Bromide intoxication—1976 literature review and case report. *Current Concepts in Psychiatry.* 2:13–20, 1976.

14. Brenner, I. Bromism: Alive and well. *American Journal of Psychiatry.* 135:857–858, 1978.

15. Stewart, R. B. Bromide intoxication from a nonprescription medication. *American Journal of Hospital Pharmacology.* 30:85–86, 1973.

16. Gault, M. H., Rudwal, T. C., & Redmond, N. I. Analgesic habits of 500 veterans: Incidence and complications of abuse. *The Canadian Medical Association Journal.* 98(13):619–626.

17. Gilles, M. A., & Skyring, A. P. The pattern and prevalence of aspirin ingestion as determined by interview of 2,921 inhabitants of Sydney. *The Medical Journal of Australia.* 1:974–979, 1972.

18. George, A. Survey of drug use in a Sydney suburb. *The Medical Journal of Australia.* 2:233–237, 1972.

19. Schuckit, M. A., & Moore, M. A. Drug problems in the elderly. In O. J. Kaplan (Ed.), *Psychopathology in the Aging.* New York: Academic Press, 1979.

20. Darlington, R. C. Laxative products. In APhA Project Staff (Eds.), *Handbook of Nonprescription Drugs,* 5th Ed. Washington, D.C.: American Pharmaceutical Association, 1977.

21. Walker, C. A. Stimulant products. In APhA Project Staff (Eds.), *Handbook of Nonprescription Drugs,* 5th Ed. Washington, D.C.: American Pharmaceutical Association, 1977.

CHAPTER 11

Multidrug Misuse

11.1. INTRODUCTION

11.1.1. General Comments

The format of this chapter differs slightly from the rest of the text in order to place the emphasis on the major types of drug interactions.

11.1.2. Problems of Definition and Classification

Investigators distinguish between *polydrug* and *multidrug* use. The former, by convention, indicates use of more than one psychoactive substance, *not including opiates*, while multidrug use is the less restrictive use of two psychoactive substances other than alcohol, nicotine, caffeine, or prescribed medications.[1] Although most polydrug clinics exclude individuals who have difficulties related to opiates,[1] the recognition that many people who primarily use multiple drugs may also casually use opiates leads me to use the less restrictive *multidrug* term here.

Abuse of multiple drugs can be further classified from a variety of clinical perspectives, none of which has been proved to be better than the others.

1. First, it is possible to divide users by the *type of drug* taken:

   a. Those who regularly abuse *narcotics* who can be subdivided into:

      i. Those who use only narcotics.
      ii. Those who use narcotics and alcohol, as well as other psychoactive substances when available.
      iii. Those who use other drugs only during methadone maintenance or when narcotics are unavailable.

b. Those who primarily abuse *alcohol* and occasionally turn to other drugs of misuse.

c. Users of *hallucinogens, stimulants,* and/or *depressants,* with or without alcohol, who do not take narcotics.

2. Another, somewhat overlapping subdivision, is based on *drug patterns*[2,3]:

a. Those who are dependent on one drug and use other drugs only when they are easily available.

b. Those who are dependent on one drug and only use other drugs when the primary substance is not available.

c. The people who prefer one drug but take others to decrease the side effects of the first.

d. Those who abuse different drugs at different times of the day, for example, stimulants in the morning, antianxiety drugs during the day, and hypnotics at night.

e. Last, those who have no drug preference but take whatever is available.

3. Of course, within any of these patterns, one must also consider:

a. The influence of prior psychiatric disorders (primary versus secondary drug abuse as described for alcohol in Section 3.1.2.3.).

b. The frequency and amount of drug misuse.

c. Whether drugs are taken intravenously or orally.

d. Whether the person is a middle-class individual usually obtaining substances from a physician or is more actively involved in a street culture.

The treatment and prognosis for individuals evidencing different patterns of multiple-drug misuse or with different psychiatric or social backgrounds may vary markedly. Thus, all of these considerations must be taken into account.

11.1.3. The Natural History of Multidrug Misuse

The ages of first use and misuse and the pattern of drug intake vary among groups. For example, a person with an antisocial personality[4] utilizes drugs as part of a larger antisocial picture—drugs are almost "incidental" to his life pattern.[5] Also, natural histories differ with the immediate environment, as exemplified by the ubiquitous availability of most drugs of abuse in urban ghettos versus middle-class suburbs. In addition, the changing views of society might be expected to have great impact on use and abuse patterns, as seen regarding marijuana.

With these caveats in mind, it is still possible to make some generalizations about likely patterns of misuse. In Western society, youth begin drug experiences with caffeine, nicotine, and alcohol. If they go on to use other substances, the next drug is likely to be marijuana, followed in frequency by one of the hallucinogens, depressants, or stimulants, usually taken on an experimental basis, ingested orally, and with few serious consequences. Individuals who go on to heavier intake may graduate to intravenous drug use, with a progression to opiates, and are thus at highest risk for developing serious drug-related difficulties.

This patterning of misuse has been viewed by some investigators as an age-related clustering of drugs that does not represent a continuum or "stepping-stone" from one particular drug to another.[6] Other researchers, however, have outlined a sequential pattern of misuse, from nonuse to beer or wine, progressing to cigarettes and/or hard liquor, and then to marijuana, which may pressage the use of other drugs.[7] These studies have indicated that it is rare for an individual to proceed directly to marijuana use without prior use of beer or cigarettes. Marijuana, in turn, is seen as a step on the road to the use of other substances. One could suggest that once an individual has crossed the barrier against the use of any substance, especially any illegal substance (remembering that alcohol is usually illegal at age 18 or under), it becomes easier to take a second and third drug.[18]

11.1.4. Pharmacology

11.1.4.1. General Comments

The effects of a drug may be either increased or decreased through interactions with other drugs:

a. The effect of a drug is *decreased* when it is administered to an individual who, while *not* taking any other drug at the same time, has developed cross-tolerance to a similar drug. This can occur through metabolic tolerance (usually reflecting the increased production of the relevant metabolic enzymes in the liver) or pharmacodynamic mechanisms (where the effect of the substance on brain cells has been decreased). Thus, higher levels of the substance are needed to generate the expected clinical effects. A relevant example is the need for higher levels of anesthetics, hypnotics, antianxiety drugs, or analgesics in alcoholics.

b. The results are the opposite, however, when two drugs with similar effects are administered *concomitantly*. Here, both drugs must compete from the same enzyme systems, both in the liver and at the target cell, the latter usually occurring in the brain. The effect is *potentiation*, where, for example, the amount of depression of brain activity that occurs from the conjoint administration of two depressant drugs or a depressant and an analgesic is more than would be expected from the actions of either drug alone. The result can be an unexpected lethal overdose for the individual who has had too much to drink and decides that a few extra sleeping pills will help him rest through the night.

11.1.4.2. Some Specific Examples

Thus, the clinician should think twice before administering more than one drug to a patient. Because of the opposing effects, specific drug–drug interactions are somewhat unpredictable, underlining the dangers in multidrug misuse. However, it is possible to make some generalizations about particular types of drug combinations.

11.1.4.2.1. Depressant–Depressants

If the drugs are not used at the same time, one would expect a decreased potency of the second depressant when administered to an individual who has already developed tolerance to the first. If, however, the two depressants (e.g., alcohol and sleeping pills) are given at the same time, potentiation of respiratory depression develops, with resulting morbidity and even mortality.[9]

11.1.4.2.2. Depressants–Opiates

Even though these drugs do not have true cross-tolerance, one frequently sees a decreased efficacy of one drug when administered to an individual who has developed tolerance to the second class. Of greater clinical importance, however, is the fact that both opiates and depressants have depressing effects on the central nervous system and, thus, potentiate the actions of the other in overdose, increasing the likelihood of death.

11.1.4.2.3. Depressant–Stimulants

The concomitant use of these drugs usually decreases the level of side effects encountered with one drug alone. The dangers rest with the unpredictability of the reaction, as the CNS and metabolic systems attempt to maintain equilibrium or homeostasis in the presence of multiple drugs with opposite effects.

11.1.4.2.4. Hallucinogens–Stimulants

The similarities in clinical action and chemical structure of these two classes of drugs frequently lead to a potentiation of side effects. This possibility militates against the use of stimulants in the treatment of a hallucinogen-related toxic reaction (see Section 8.2.3.2.), as clinical symptoms may worsen, not improve.

11.1.4.2.5. Hallucinogens–Atropinic Drugs

The same generalizations hold here as for the hallucinogen–stimulant interaction, making it unwise to use antipsychotic medications, with their anticholinergic side effects, in treating patients with a hallucinogen-induced toxic reaction or an over-the-counter hyponotic or antianxiety drug overdose.

11.1.4.2.6. Marijuana–Other Drugs

Marijuana has been shown to potentiate the CNS depressing effect of alcohol,[10] and it may increase the likelihood of a flashback from hallucinogen-type drugs. While these relationships require more research, it is unwise to take marijuana concomitantly with other substances, especially alcohol, because of resulting motor incoordination and CNS depression, a problem with great implications to driving abilities.[11,12]

11.1.5. Epidemiology and Patterns of Abuse

While the extent of multiple-drug misuse is not known, it appears to be a rather common phenomenon among drug abusers. There is also anecdotal evidence that multiple-substance misuse has increased over the years.[3,13,14] This is not surprising, considering that as many as 90% of young people report the use of alcohol, almost 60% have used marijuana, and almost 20% report use of amphetamines, barbiturates, or LSD.[15]

Over one-half of the people presenting to a polydrug clinic report the use of three or more substances.[16,17] Certain individuals appear to be at especially high risk for multidrug misuse, including those with a history of psychiatric problems,[18] those "denied" access to their favorite drug (for example, subjects in methadone maintenance programs[19]), and those who deliberately use the more "exotic" substances, such as phencyclidine (PCP)[20] (see Section 8.3.). A fourth special group live in high-stress situations while separated from their families, such as the young soldiers using drugs, 70% of whom, according to one survey, persistently administer multiple substances.[17-21]

In general, multidrug users tend to be young and from middle-class backgrounds and often show some evidence of preexisting life maladjustment, which might be labeled a personality disorder.[22]

11.1.6. Establishing a Diagnosis

It is important to remember that substance abuse is a relatively common phenomenon in our society and must be considered in the differential diagnosis of a wide variety of medical and psychological problems. To review briefly, in evaluating an individual who, by past history, fits the criteria for the antisocial personality, one must note the likelihood that he/she is abusing multiple drugs. This is also probable for those who use less usually available substances, such as phencyclidine (PCP, see Section 8.3.), those on methadone maintenance programs, and those living in high-stress situations. On another level, any individual presenting to the emergency room with a drug overdose must be evaluated for the *possibility* of multiple-drug misuse, particularly any person who does not show the usual response to emergency room interventions.

11.2. EMERGENCY ROOM SITUATIONS

The most important clinical pictures seen with multiple drugs include toxic reactions (usually overdoses), drug withdrawal pictures, psychoses, and organic brain syndromes. The discussion given here is brief, as, once multiple-drug problems are indicated, treatment involves combining those procedures used for each substance alone.

11.2.1. Panic Reactions (See Section 1.6.1.)

The clinical picture, course, and treatment for panic reactions resemble those seen for any one of the substances, including marijuana, hallucinogens, stimulants, and the atropinic drugs. Treatment is as outlined in the specific drug chapters. Good examples are given in Sections 5.2.1., 7.2.1., and 12.2.

11.2.2. Flashbacks

Flashbacks are seen with the hallucinogens or marijuana, and the clinical course and treatment for recurrences after use of these drugs in combination with others is the same as outlined in Sections 6.2.3., and 7.2.3., for the individual drugs.

11.2.3. Toxic Reactions (See Sections 1.6.3., and 12.4.)

11.2.3.1. The Clinical Picture

Toxic reactions, of great clinical significance, result from the concomitant administration of two depressant-type drugs or of opiates along with depressants.

11.2.3.1.1. Multiple Depressants (See Sections 2.2.3., and 4.2.3.)

Multiple-depressant overdosage is complex because the depth of respiratory depression and the length of severe toxicity is difficult to predict. However, the clinical manifestations are those described for CNS depressants and for alcohol.

11.2.3.1.2. Depressants–Opiates (See Sections 2.2.3., and 6.2.3.)

The concomitant administration of opiates and depressants results in unpredictable vital signs, reflexes, and pupillary reactions, along with fluctuation between stupor and semialertness.[2] The specific symptoms are combinations of those reported for the CNS depressants and opiates.

11.2.3.2. Treatment

11.2.3.2.1. Multiple Depressants

For mixed-depressant toxic reactions, treatment is outlined in Section 2.2.3., including acute life-preserving steps and use of general life supports, relying on the body to detoxify the substances. Dialysis or diuresis should be reserved for extremely toxic cases.

11.2.3.2.2. Depressants–Opiates

In the instance of combined opiate and CNS-depressant overdose, acute emergency procedures (e.g., airway, cardiac status, etc.) are again followed. Naloxone (Narcan) is administered at doses of 0.4 mg IM or IV, with repeat doses given every 5 minutes for the first 15 minutes and every several hours thereafter, as needed, for control of respiratory depression and the degree of stupor. These procedures are outlined in Sections 2.2.3., and 6.2.3.

11.2.3.2.3. Other Combinations

The treatment of other drug combinations is symptomatic in nature and follows treatment procedures outlined in the relevant drug chapters. It is worthwhile to note the importance of physostigmine when atropinic drugs (such as the over-the-counter hypnotics and antianxiety drugs or benztropine [Cogentin]) are involved (Section 10.2.4.2.).

11.2.4. Psychoses (See Section 1.6.4.)

The drug-induced psychoses seen with stimulants (Section 5.2.4.) and CNS depressants (Sections 2.2.4., and 4.2.4.) are evanescent pictures, disappearing with general supportive care. Little, if any, information is available on the psychosis produced by multiple administration of these substances.

11.2.5. Organic Brain Syndrome (See Section 1.6.5.)

Any drug in high enough doses can cause confusion and disorientation, the hallmarks of an organic brain syndrome. In drug combinations, one can expect this clinical picture to be evanescent and should follow the general treatment plans outlined in the individual chapters. However, it is wise to remember that with multiple drugs, the course is unpredictable, and it is probable that the patient will be impaired for a longer time than would be expected for either drug alone.

11.2.6. Withdrawal from Multiple Drugs (See Section 1.6.6.)

The most common multiple-drug withdrawal pictures are those seen following the concomitant abuse of multiple depressants, depressants and stimulants, or multiple addictions to opiates and depressant drugs.

11.2.6.1. Clinical Picture

11.2.6.1.1. Multiple Depressants

The depressant withdrawal syndrome, described in Section 2.2.6., is similar for all CNS-depressant drugs; however, a higher incidence of convulsions is seen with hypnotics or antianxiety drugs than with alcohol. The latency of onset and length of the acute withdrawal syndrome roughly parallels the half-life of the drugs, ranging from relatively short periods of time for alcohol to much longer withdrawals for drugs such as chlordiazepoxide (Librium) and phenobarbital.

11.2.6.1.2. Depressants–Stimulants (See Sections 2.2.6., and 5.2.6.)

The withdrawal from depressants and stimulants more closely follows the CNS-depressant withdrawal paradigm but includes greater levels of sadness, paranoia, and lethargy than would be expected with depressants alone.

11.2.6.1.3. Depressants–Opiates

The individual withdrawing from depressants and opiates usually demonstrates an opiate withdrawal syndrome (Section 6.2.6.), but convulsions and confusion may be important parts of the picture (see Sections 2.2.6., and 4.2.6.).

11.2.6.1.4. Other Combinations

Withdrawal pictures from other classes of drugs either have not been proved to exist or have low levels of clinical significance; therefore, multiple withdrawal syndromes of drugs other than depressants, stimulants, and opiates will not be discussed here.

11.2.6.2. Treatment

11.2.6.2.1. Multiple Depressants

Adequate therapy for physical addiction to multiple depressants follows the guidelines outlined in Section 2.2.6., with the added caveat that the time course of withdrawal is unpredictable.

1. Thus, it is unwise to decrease the level of administered CNS depressant at a rate faster than 10% a day, taking special care to reinstitute the last day's dose at any sign of impending serious withdrawal.

2. It is usually possible to carry out a smooth withdrawal from multiple CNS depressants by administering only one of those depressant drugs to the point where symptoms are abolished on Day 1.

11.2.6.2.2. Depressants–Stimulants

In the case of multiple addiction to depressants and stimulants, it is the depressant withdrawal syndrome that produces the greatest amount of discomfort and is the most life-threatening (Section 2.2.6.). Thus, while recognizing an intensification of some of the symptoms, it is best to proceed with the mode of treatment for depressant withdrawal.

11.2.6.2.3. Depressants–Opiates

1. In the case of addiction to CNS depressants and to opiates, it is advisable to administer both an opiate and a CNS depressant, as outlined in Sections 2.2.6., and 6.2.6., until withdrawal symptoms have been abolished.

2. Most authors then recommend stabilization with the opiate (Section 6.2.6.), while the depressant is withdrawn at 10% a day (Section 2.2.6.).

3. After the depressant withdrawal is completed, opiate withdrawal can then proceed (Section 6.2.6.).[2,23,24]

11.2.7. Medical Problems

Concomitant administration of two substances over an extended period of time does, in all likelihood, increase the risk of development of medical consequences. However, the specific problems depend upon the specific drugs involved, as well as the individual's age, preexisting medical disorders, and concomitant nutritional status and experience of stress. When treating a patient misusing multiple drugs, the clinician should review the sections on medical problems in each of the relevant chapters.

One special problem is seen in those individuals whose drug abuse has occurred secondary to attempts at controlling pain, usually by misusing depressants or analgesics on a doctor's prescription. Pain syndromes that are unresponsive to usual measures (frequently back pain and chronic headache) are very difficult to treat and not at all well understood. It is important to gather a history of any addiction and of concomitant medical complaints in evaluating any drug misuser. Following withdrawal, these identified individuals can be included as part of a polydrug or individual drug program, but they will probably also require additional care, such as that offered in specialized pain clinics.[25,26]

REFERENCES

1. Kaufman, E. The abuse of multi drugs. 1. Definition, classification, and extent of problem. *American Journal of Drug and Alcohol Abuse.* 3(2):272–292, 1976.
2. Cohen, S. Polydrug abuse. *Drug Abuse and Alcoholism Newsletter* 5(2), 1976. San Diego: Vista Hill Foundation.
3. National Clearinghouse for Drug Abuse Information. *Polydrug Use: An Annotated Bibliography.* Rockville, Md.: National Institute on Drug Abuse, 1975.
4. Woodruff, R. A., Goodwin, D. W., & Guze, S. B. *Psychiatric Diagnosis.* New York: Oxford University Press, 1974.
5. Schuckit, M. A. Alcoholism and sociopathy-diagnostic confusion. *Quarterly Journal of Studies on Alcohol.* 34(1):157–164, 1973.
6. Hamburg, B. A., Kraemer, H. C., & Jahnke, W. A hierarchy of drug use in adolescence: Behavioral and attitudinal. *American Journal of Psychiatry.* 132(11):1155–1164, 1975.
7. Kandel, D. Antecedents of adolescent initiation into stages of drug use. In D. Kandel (Ed.), *Longitudinal Research on Drug Use.* Washington, D.C.: Hemisphere Publishing, 1978, Chapter 3.
8. Gould, L. C., & Kleber, H. D. Changing patterns of multiple drug use among applicants to a multimodality drug treatment program. *Archives of General Psychiatry.* 31:408–413, 1974.
9. Cohen, S. Psychotropic drug interactions. *Drug Abuse and Alcoholism Newsletter.* 6(6). San Diego: Vista Hill Foundation, 1977.

10. Siemens, A. J., Kalant, H., & Khanna, J. M. Effects of cannabis on pentobarbital induced sleeping time and pentobarbital metabolsim in the rat. *Biochemistry Pharmacology.* 23:477–489, 1974.

11. Janowsky, D. S., Meacham, M. P., Blane, J. D., *et al.* Simulated flying performance after marihuana intoxication. *Aviation, Space, and Environmental Medicine.* 47:124–128, 1976.

12. Whitehead, P. C., & Ferrence, R. G. Alcohol and other drugs related to young drivers' traffic accident involvement. *Journal of Safety Research.* 8(2):65–72, 1976.

13. Simpson, D. D., & Sells, S. B. Patterns of multiple drug abuse: 1969–1971. *The International Journal of the Addictions.* 9(2):301–314, 1974.

14. Blackford, L. Student drug use surveys—San Mateo County, California, 1968–1975. San Mateo, Calif.: Department of Public Health and Welfare, June 6, 1975.

16. Grant, I., & Mohns, L. Chronic cerebral effects of alcohol and drug abuse. *The International Journal of the Addictions.* 10(5):883–920, 1975.

17. Cook, R. F., Hostetter, R. S., & Ramsay, D. A. Patterns of illicit drug use in the Army. *American Journal of Psychiatry.* 132(10):1013–1017, 1975.

18. Fischer, D. E., Halikas, J. A., Baker, J. W., *et al.* Frequency and patterns of drug abuse in psychiatric patients. *Diseases of the Nervous System.* 36:550–553, 1975.

19. Green, J., & Jaffe, J. H. Alcohol and opiate dependence. A review. *Journal of Studies on Alcohol.* 38(7):1274–1293, 1977.

20. Schuckit, M. A., & Morrissey, E. R. Propoxyphene and phencyclidine (PCP) use in adolescents. *Journal of Clinical Psychiatry.* 39(1):7–13, 1978.

21. Callan, J. P., & Patterson, C. P. Patterns of drug abuse among military inductees. *American Journal of Psychiatry.* 130:260–264, 1973.

22. Prichep, L. S., Cohen, M., Kaplan, J., *et al.* Psychiatric evaluation services to court referred drug users. *American Journal of Drug & Alcohol Abuse.* 2(2):197–213, 1975.

23. Sapira, J. D., & Cherubin, C. E. Drug abuse. A guide for the clinician. *Excerpta Medica.* Amsterdam: American Elsevier, 1975.

24. Smith, D. E., & Wesson, D. R. Phenobarbital technique for treatment of barbiturate dependence. *Archives of General Psychiatry.* 24:56–60, 1971.

25. Halpern, L. M. Treating pain with drugs. *Minnesota Medicine.* 57:176–185, 1974.

26. Sternbach, R. A. *Pain: Psychophysiologic Analysis.* New York: Academic Press, 1968.

CHAPTER 12

Emergency Problems: A Rapid Overview

12.1. INTRODUCTION

12.1.1. Comments

The goal of this chapter is to teach some general guidelines for drug emergencies. The material is presented from a different perspective than is true of the rest of the text. I have approached the problem from the standpoint of patient symptoms, assuming a situation where you do not know the specific drug involved. The chapter is divided into topic areas similar to those already presented, with emergent situations ranging from panic to medical problems.

12.1.2. Some General Rules

1. By common sense, first address life-threatening problems, then gather a more substantial history and carry out other patient care procedures, and finally, plan disposition and future treatment.[1,2]

2. Avoid giving additional medications whenever possible.[1] Administration of additional drugs to an individual with a drug-related problem can result in unpredictable drug–drug interactions, made all the worse by the high level of arousal usually demonstrated by the patient. However, when there is good reason for administering medications, it is important that they be given in doses adequate to produce clinical affects.

3. It is always important to establish a complete history by gathering information from the patient *and an additional resource person,* usually a spouse. For a patient who is stuporous or out of contact with reality, the patient's belongings might contain the names of individuals able to provide accurate information.

12.1.3. An Introduction to Specific Emergency Problems[3,4]

Table 12.1 gives some helpful symptoms and signs that can be used in making an educated guess as to which drug was taken and the future course of problems. I must emphasize that this table allows you only to establish a *guesstimate*. The chart has not been tested in controlled investigations and therefore can be used as nothing more than a guideline.

An example of the use of this table would be an individual who comes to you with decreased respiration and pinpoint pupils: one of the first things to be considered is a toxic opiate overdose. A second example is an individual who comes with an elevated temperature and warm, dry skin with fixed, dilated pupils: this is probably a toxic reaction involving an atropinelike anticholinergic drug.

I will now proceed with a discussion of each of the major emergency

Table 12.1
A Rough Guide to Symptoms in Drug Reactions

Symptom or sign	Reaction type	Possible Drugs
Vital signs		
Blood pressure		
Increase	Toxic	Stimulants or LSD
Decrease	Withdrawal	Depressants
Pulse		
Increase	Toxic	Stimulants
	Withdrawal	Depressants
Body temperature		
Irregular	Toxic	Solvents or stimulants
Increase	Toxic	Atropine-type, stimulants, or LSD
Decrease	Withdrawal	Opiates or depressants
Repirations		
Decrease	Toxic	Opiates or depressants
Head		
Eyes		
Pupils		
Pinpoint	Toxic	Opiates
Dilated, reactive	Toxic	Hallucinogens, withdrawal, opiates
Dilated, sluggish	Toxic	Glutethimide or stimulants
Dilated, unreactive	Toxic	Atropine-type
Sclera		
Injected (bloodshot)	Toxic	Marijuana or solvents
Nystagmus	Toxic	Depressants
Tearing	Withdrawal	Opiates

Symptom or sign	Reaction type	Possible drugs
Nose		
Runny (rhinorrhea)	Withdrawal	Opiates
Dry	Toxic	Atropine-type
Ulcers in membranes or septum	Chronic use	Cocaine
Skin		
Warm, dry	Toxic	Atropine-type
Warm, moist	Toxic	Stimulants
Needle marks	Chronic use	Opiates, stimulants, or depressants
Gooseflesh	Toxic	LSD
	Withdrawal	Opiates
Rash over mouth or nose	Toxic	Solvents
Speech		
Slow, not slurred	Toxic	Opiates
Slow, slurred	Toxic	Depressants
Rapid	Toxic	Stimulants
Hands		
Fine tremor	Toxic	Stimulants or hallucinogens
	Withdrawal	Opiates
Coarse tremor	Withdrawal	Depressants
Neurological		
Reflexes		
Increased	Toxic	Stimulants
Decreased	Toxic	Depressants
Convulsions	Toxic	Stimulants, codeine, propoxyphene, methaqualude
Lungs		
Pulmonary edema	Toxic	Opiates or depressants

room situations, first giving a definition, than making some generalizations about the drug state and reviewing some of the drugs that might be involved. The reader is encouraged to return to chapters dealing with specific drugs for more in-depth discussions.

12.2. PANIC REACTIONS (See Sections 1.6.1.)

12.2.1. Clinical Picture

The panic reaction is identified by a patient's presenting with a high level of anxiety, usually expressing fears that he is losing control, is going crazy, is having a heart attack, or has done damage to his body. He may give a drug history and is able to maintain contact with reality in a highly structured environment. The history usually demonstrates that the patient is a naive user and that other individuals have taken the same amount of drug with no serious effects. This state is usually a benign, self-limited, emotional overreaction to usual drug effects.[5]

12.2.2. Differential Diagnosis

Panic reactions most frequently occur with drugs that stimulate the user and change the level of consciousness: *hallucinogens, cannibis,* or *stimulants.* It is important to rule out physical disease (e.g., a genuine heart attack or a hyperthyroid state) and to consider possible psychiatric pictures, such as anxiety neurosis, obsessive neurosis, or a phobic neurosis.[6]

12.2.3. Treatment

The cornerstone of treatment is reassurance, education about the drug effects, and time.
1. Carry out a quick physical examination.
2. Gather a history of recent events.
3. Give reassurance, talk to the patient as frequently as possible, and help him to orient to time, place, and person. It is best to place the patient in a quiet room, with friends or relatives available to help "talk him down."
4. For those individuals showing a lability in vital signs, bed rest is important, with carefully monitored blood pressure and pulse.
5. Avoid additional medication, but where needed, I would suggest a benzodiazepine (e.g., diazepam [Valium] at doses of 15–30 mg) given either orally or, if absolutely necessary, intramuscularly. These doses can be repeated every 1–2 hours as needed, keeping the dose as low as possible.

12.3. FLASHBACKS (See Section 1.6.2.)

12.3.1. Clinical Picture

This drug-induced state involves a recurrence of feelings of intoxication some time after the initial drug effects have worn off. This is a benign, self-limited condition that rarely, if ever, represents a serious physical threat.

12.3.2. Differential Diagnosis

Flashbacks are seen primarily with *marijuana* and the *hallucinogens*. It is, however, also important to take time to rule out the possibility of underlying psychiatric disorders, especially schizophrenia or affective disorder,[6] or an organic brain syndrome.

12.3.3. Treatment

The approach to this condition is straightforward reassurance and education.[5] If the person does not respond to reassurance, he may be administered an antianxiety drug such as diazepam (Valium) in doses of 10–20 mg orally, repeated as needed.[5]

12.4. TOXIC REACTIONS (See Section 1.6.3.)

12.4.1. Clinical Picture

In this instance, the individual has ingested more than the usual amount of a substance and presents with an overdose. To allow for generalizations, I have, somewhat arbitrarily, distinguished in this text between a *toxic overdose*, with unstable vital signs predominating; a *psychosis*, with hallucinations and delusions in an alert individual; and an *organic brain syndrome*, where the major symptomatology is confusion and disorientation. However, the high level of overlap between these syndromes must be noted.

12.4.2. Differential Diagnosis

The serious overdoses are most likely to be seen with drugs that depress the CNS, such as *opiates*, PCP, and *depressants*. Because the treatments for the toxic reactions of these drugs differ slightly, it is important to identify the drug involved.

There are no major psychiatric syndromes that mimic the overdose, with the possible exception of a catatoniclike stupor seen with serious depression,[6] but medical disorders that can cause coma (e.g., hypoglycemia or severe electrolyte abnormalities) must be considered.

12.4.3. Treatment

Definitive treatment of shocklike states is complex and requires precise knowledge that is beyond the scope of this text. Briefly, it is necessary to address acute life supports and then provide general patient care, allowing the body to metabolize the drug ingested.

12.4.3.1. Acute Life-Saving Measures (See References 9–17.)

1. Establish the vital signs.
2. Assure adequate ventilation. This includes:

   a. Straightening the head.
   b. Removing any obstructions from the throat.
   c. Carrying out artificial respiration, if necessary.
   d. Doing tracheal intubation, if necessary (use an inflatable cuff tube, if at all possible, to allow for gastric lavage).
   e. Establishing the patient on a respirator, if necessary. Use 10–12 respirations per minute, avoiding oxygen, as this may decrease spontaneous respirations.
   f. Maintaining an adequate circulatory state. This includes very briefly:

      i. If the heart is stopped, use external chest massage and administer intracardiac adrenaline.
      ii. If there's evidence of cardiac fibrillation, use a defibrillator.
      iii. If inadequate circulation is evident, an intravenous drip of 50 ml of sodium bicarbonate (3.75 g) should be used to treat the acidic state.

3. Carry out a quick physical examination to rule out serious bleeding, life-threatening trauma, etc.
4. Start an IV:

   a. Use a large-gauge needle.
   b. Use restraints, if necessary, to make sure that the needle will stay in place.
   c. Use a slow IV drip until the need for intravenous fluids has been established.[9]

5. Draw blood for chemical analysis:

   a. 10 cc, at a minimum, is needed for a toxicologic screen.
   b. 30–40 cc is necessary for the usual blood count, electrolytes, blood sugar, and BUN.

6. If there is any chance that the individual is hypoglycemic, administer 50 cc of 50% glucose IV.
7. An EKG or rhythm strip is especially important because of the cardiac irregularities that may be seen with nonbarbituate hypnotics.[10,11]
8. For recent ingestions, carry out gastric lavage[10]:

   a. Do not do this until the heart rate is stable, to avoid inducing a clinically significant vagal response.

    b. If the patient is not awake, carry out lavage only after tracheal intubation with a tube with an inflatable cuff to avoid aspiration.

    c. Gastric lavage is carried out only on individuals who have taken drugs orally within the last 4–6 or, at most, 12 hours.

    d. After evacuating the stomach, administer a saline lavage until the returned fluid looks clear.

    e. Consider administering activated charcoal or castor oil (60 ml) to help stop absorption for oral overdoses—castor oil is especially important for lipid-soluble substances such as glutethimide (Doriden).

    9. Collect urine if possible—this may require catheterizing the bladder. Send 50 ml of the urine for a toxicologic screen.[3]

    10. If the patient's blood pressure has not responded, you may use plasma expanders or pressors as for any shocklike state, taking care to titrate the needed dose and being aware of any potentially life-threatening drug interactions.

    11. If there is a chance that the overdose includes an opiate, administer a test dose of naloxone (Narcan)[12] in doses of 0.4–0.8 mg (1–2 ml) IM or IV, as discussed earlier (Section 6.2.3.2.). However, it is important to beware of precipitating a severe opiate withdrawal syndrome—this would usually be treated with reassurance and readministration of a mild analgesic, such as propoxyphene (Darvon), or with methadone (Section 6.2.6.2.).

    12. If the overdose appears to involve an atropinelike (anticholinergic) drug as indicated by a rapid heart rate, dry skin and mouth, a rash, etc., consider giving physostignine, 1–4 mg, by slow IV injection.

12.4.3.2. Subacute Treatment

    1. Establish the vital signs every 15 minutes for at least the first 4 hours; then monitor carefully (perhaps every 2–4 hours) over the next 24–48 hours, even if the patient's condition is improved. Many of the substances (e.g., the fat-soluble hypnotics like glutethimide [Doriden] or ethchlorvynol [Placidyl]) clear from the plasma temporarily and are then rereleased from fat stores, causing severe reintoxication after the patient has apparently improved. Also, for opiate overdoses, the antagonists are active only for a relatively short period after administration.

    2. Carry out a thorough physical examination, with special emphasis on the status and changes in neurological signs.[9,11]

    3. Gather an intensive history from the patient and a resource person, such as the spouse.

4. Establish a flow sheet to monitor vital signs, medications, fluid intake, fluid output, etc.[9]

5. Establish a baseline weight that can be used as a guide to fluid balance.[10]

6. Dialysis or diuresis is rarely needed[13]:

   a. If you choose to carry out diuresis, you may use furosemide (Lasix) in doses of 40–100 mg, administered regularly to maintain a urinary output of approximately 250 ml per hour. Of course, it is very important to replace electrolytes and fluids.[10]

   b. Diuresis can also be carried out through the careful administration of enough intravenous fluids to maintain a urinary output in excess of 200 ml/hour using half-normal saline with potassium supplementation (Section 2.2.3.2.).

   c. Dialysis is effective for almost all nonbarbiturate sedatives.[10] If available, hemodialysis is preferable to peritoneal dialysis, as the former tends to be more efficient and has less chance of decreasing respiration.

   Indications for dialysis include: severe intoxication with markedly abnormal vital signs, report of probable ingestion of a lethal dose of the drug, blood levels of the drug in the lethal dose range, impaired excretion or metabolism of the drugs due to liver or kidney damage, progressive clinical deterioration, prolonged coma, underlying lung disease, etc. Once again, it is important to emphasize that most overdose patients will recover completely without dialysis or diuresis.

7. Avoid administering any medications unless absolutely necessary.

8. If the patient is comatose, take the steps necessary for adequate care, including careful management of electrolytes and fluids, eye care, frequent turning of the patient, careful tracheal toilet, etc.

12.5. PSYCHOSIS (See Section 1.6.4.)

12.5.1. Clinical Picture

Psychosis is a loss of contact with reality, which, as discussed in this text, occurs in the midst of a clear sensorium. The patient usually presents with hallucinations (most frequently auditory) and/or delusions (usually persecutory). Although clinically very dramatic, this is usually a self-limited problem, running its course within a matter of days to a week for most drugs (exceptions are STP and PCP).

12.5.2. Differential Diagnosis

Any psychiatric disorder capable of producing a psychotic picture, especially schizophrenia, mania, an organic brain syndrome, or depression, must be considered as part of the differential diagnosis.[6] The drugs most frequently involved in psychoses are *alcohol*, the other *CNS depressants, stimulants*, and *PCP*.

12.5.3. Treatment

The major goal is to protect the patient from harming himself or others, or from carrying out acts that would be embarrassing or would cause later difficulties. At the same time, it is important to review problems adequately to rule out other serious medical and psychiatric disorders. The patient presenting with a hallucinating/delusional state, therefore, usually requires hospitalization until the delusions clear.

12.6. ORGANIC BRAIN SYNDROME (See Section 1.6.5.)

12.6.1. Clinical Picture

The organic state can be caused by high doses of any drug and consists of confusion and disorientation along with decreased general mental functioning. This reaction may be accompanied by illusions (misinterpretation of real stimuli, such as shadows or machinery sounds), hallucinations (usually visual or tactile), or delusions.

12.6.2. Differential Diagnosis

Any drug can cause an organic brain syndrome, but in clinical practice this problem is most likely to be seen with *CNS depressants, atropine-type drugs, solvents, stimulants*, and *phencyclidine* (PCP).[18,19]

Whenever organicity is observed, it is important to consider the possibility of acute or chronic brain damage, trauma, vitamin deficiency, or serious medical problems that might disrupt electrolytes. If these medical disorders are overlooked, a life-threatening condition can ensue.

12.6.3. Treatment

Treatment consists of general life supports. Because this problem is either a minor toxic reaction or the early stage of a serious overdose, treatment is identical to that outlined above in the relevant toxic reaction. Although most organicities disappear within a matter of hours to days, some secondary OBS pictures caused by vitamin deficiencies or traumas can take many months to clear.

12.7. DRUG WITHDRAWAL STATES (See Section 1.6.6.)

12.7.1. Clinical Picture

The sudden cessation or rapid decrease in intake of any of the drugs capable of producing physical dependence can result in the withdrawal state. This, simplistically, is manifested by anxiety, a heightened drive to obtain the drug, a flulike syndrome, and physiological symptoms that are usually in the direction opposite to those expected with intoxication.

Withdrawal is rarely life-threatening, with the possible exception of CNS depressants, unless the patient is allowed to go through it in a seriously impaired physical state.

12.7.2. Differential Diagnosis

It is important to determine whether the withdrawal state is related to *stimulants, depressants,* or *opiate analgesics,* since the specific treatments differ greatly. It is also necessary to rule out the physiological disorders that can result in a flulike syndrome and to implement proper medical treatment.

12.7.3. Treatment

In addition to recognizing and treating all concomitant medical disorders, offer reassurance, rest, and good nutrition.

1. Carry out a good physical examination, taking special care to rule out infections, hepatitis, subdural hematomas, heart failure, and electrolyte abnormalities. A patient entering withdrawal with impaired physical functioning has a markedly increased chance of dying during the withdrawal. Also, if any physiological abnormality is overlooked at the inception of withdrawal, it may be difficult, as the absence syndrome progresses, to tell whether abnormal vital signs are a response to the withdrawal or represent other physical pathology.[20,21]

2. Specific treatment of the withdrawal depends upon recognition of the fact that symptoms have developed because the drug of addiction has been stopped *too quickly.* Therefore, the basic paradigm of treatment is giving enough of the drug of addiction (or one to which the individual has cross-tolerance) to greatly diminish withdrawal symptoms on Day 1. This drug is then decreased by 10–20% of the initial day's dosage each day over the subsequent 5–10 days.

REFERENCES

1. Greenblatt, D. J., & Shader, R. I. Drug abuse and the emergency room physician. *American Journal of Psychiatry.* 131(5):559–562, 1974.
2. Chapel, J. L. Emergency room treatment of the drug-abusing patient. *American Journal of Psychiatry.* 130(3):257–259, 1973.
3. Dimijian, G. G. Differential diagnosis of emergency drug reactions. In P. G. Bourne (Ed.), *A Treatment Manual for Acute Drug Abuse Emergencies.* Washington, D.C.: U.S. Government Printing Office, 1974, pp. 1–7.
4. Rubin, P. E., & Cluff, L. E. Differential diagnosis of emergency drug reactions. In P. G. Bourne (Ed.), *A Treatment Manual for Acute Drug Abuse Emergencies.* Washington, D.C.: U.S. Government Printing Office, 1974, pp. 8–10.
5. Ungerleiter, J. T., & Frank, I. M. Management of acute panic reactions and flashbacks resulting from LSD ingestion. In P. G. Bourne (Ed.), *A Treatment Manual for Acute Drug Abuse Emergencies.* Washington, D.C.: U.S. Government Printing Office, 1974, pp. 73–76.
6. Woodruff, R. A., Goodwin, D. W., & Guze, S. B. *Psychiatric Diagnosis.* New York: Oxford University Press, 1974.
7. Schoichet, R. Emergency treatment of acute adverse reactions to hallucinogenic drugs. In P. G. Bourne (Ed.), *A Treatment Manual for Acute Drug Abuse Emergencies.* Washington, D.C.: U.S. Government Printing Office, 1974, pp. 80–82.
8. Cohen, S. The witches' brews. In S. Cohen (Ed.), *Drug Abuse and Alcoholism Newsletter.* 7(2):1–4, 1978.
9. Setter, J. G. Emergency treatment of acute barbiturate intoxication. In P. G. Bourne (Ed.), *A Treatment Manual for Acute Drug Abuse Emergencies.* Washington, D.C.: U.S. Government Printing Office, 1974, pp. 49–53.
10. Cronin, R. J., Klingler, E. L., Avasthi, P. S., et al. The treatment of nonbarbiturate sedative overdosage. In P. G. Bourne (Ed.), *A Treatment Manual for Acute Drug Abuse Emergencies.* Washington, D.C.: U.S. Government Printing Office, 1974, pp. 58–61.
11. Afifi, A. A., Sacks, S. T., Liu, V. Y., et al. Accumulative prognostic index for patients with barbiturate, glutethimide and meprobamate intoxication. *New England Journal of Medicine.* 285:1497–1502, 1971.
12. Waldron, V. D., Klimt, C. R., & Seibel, J. E. Methadone overdose treated with naloxone infusion. *Journal of the American Medical Association.* 225(1):53, 1973.
13. Wright, N., & Roscoe, P. Acute glutethimide poisoning. *Journal of the American Medical Association.* 214(9):1704–1706, 1970.
14. Greene, M. H., & DuPont, R. L. The treatment of acute heroin toxicity. In P. G. Bourne (Ed.), *A Treatment Manual for Acute Drug Abuse Emergencies.* Washington, D.C.: U.S. Government Printing Office, 1974, pp. 11–16.
15. Kleber, H. D. The treatment of acute heroin toxicity. In P. G. Bourne (Ed.), *A Treatment Manual for Acute Drug Abuse Emergencies.* Washington, D.C.: U.S. Government Printing Office, 1974, pp. 17–21.
16. Ellinwood, E. H., Jr. Emergency treatment of acute adverse reactions to CNS stimulants. In P. G. Bourne (Ed.), *A Treatment Manual for Acute Drug Abuse Emergencies.* Washington, D.C.: U.S. Government Printing Office, 1974, pp. 63–67.

17. Tinklenberg, J. R. The treatment of acute amphetamine psychosis. In P. G. Bourne (Ed.), *A Treatment Manual for Acute Drug Abuse Emergencies.* Washington, D.C.: U.S. Government Printing Office, 1974, pp. 68–72.

18. Lewis, P. W., & Patterson, D. W. Acute and chronic effects of the voluntary inhalation of certain commercial volatile solvents by juveniles. *Journal of Drug Issues. Spring:* 162–175, 1974.

19. Schuckit, M. A., & Morrissey, E. R. Propoxyphene and phencyclidine (PCP) use in adolescents. *Journal of Clinical Psychiatry. 39*(1):7–13, 1978.

20. Preskorn, S. H., & Denner, L. J. Benzodiazepines and withdrawal psychosis. A report of three cases. *Journal of the American Medical Association. 237*(1):36–38, 1977.

21. De Bard, M. L. Diazepam withdrawal syndrome. *American Journal of Psychiatry 136*:104–105, 1979.

Rehabilitation

13.1. INTRODUCTION

This chapter serves as an introduction to the concept of rehabilitation for alcoholism and drug abuse rather than a definitive discussion of all aspects of care. It can be read for general knowledge, for guidelines for appropriate referral of patients, as a framework for the critical evaluation of programs, or as a basis for development of your own treatment efforts. I will first present a series of general rules that (with modifications) fit rehabilitation for all substance misusers. This is followed by a discussion of guidelines specifically tailored to particular drug approaches.

13.1.1. Some General Rules

The same basic guidelines apply to all types of rehabilitation efforts with substance misusers.

13.1.1.1. Justify Your Actions

Our patients, coming to see us in the midst of crises, may be prepared to "do almost anything" to make things improve. All substance-abuse problems tend to fluctuate naturally in intensity, with the result that one can see improvement with time alone. There is also a considerable rate of "spontaneous remission" with no intervention at all. The key questions to be addressed in judging any treatment are: "Did the improvement occur *because* of the treatment?" and "Were the therapeutic efforts those with the greatest chance for success?"[1] The therapist must constantly justify his actions, both in a financial cost–benefit framework and in a manner that considers patient and staff time, physical or emotional dangers to the patient, and the trauma of separation from job and family.

13.1.1.2. Know the Natural Course of the Disorder

It is only through knowledge of the probable course of drug misuse that one can make adequate treatment plans.[2,3]

13.1.1.3. Guard against Overzealous Acceptance of New Treatments

Most treatment efforts "make sense" in some theoretical framework; and most patients improve, and many get "well," no matter what treatment is used. Therefore, demand good controlled investigations before accepting newer treatment approaches as valid.

13.1.1.4. Keep It Simple

In evaluating treatment efforts or accepting new therapies, a sensible approach is to stay with the least costly, least potentially harmful, and simplest maneuvers until there are good data to justify more complex procedures.

13.1.1.5. Apply Objective Diagnostic Criteria

It is not enough to accept a patient into a program because he/she presents at the door of a treatment center. In order to apply knowledge of the natural course and predict future problems, as well as to justify treatment efforts, standard diagnostic criteria must be applied to each patient.[4] An individual may, however, be labeled "ill but undiagnosed" and given a tenuous set of working diagnoses; may be given a "probable" diagnosis and treated as if he/she had a definite disorder but with extra care taken to reevaluate the label at a future date; or may be given a definite diagnosis. Of course, all patients must be evaluated for major preexisting psychiatric disorders requiring treatment or affecting prognosis.

13.1.1.6. Establish Realistic Goals

In substance misuse we rarely achieve "dramatic cures." I attempt to maximize the chances for recovery, to encourage abstinence at an earlier age than might have been achieved with no therapeutic intervention, to offer good medical care, to help the people close to the patient better understand what is going on, and to educate patients so they can make their own decisions about treatment goals. Although health care practitioners can and must offer their best efforts, the patient's motivation and level of "readiness" for recovery have a great impact on outcome.

13.1.1.7. Know the Goals of Your Patients

In establishing patient goals, it is important to understand the patient's reasons for entering treatment: Was it to detox only? To meet a crisis? or actually, To aim at long-term abstinence?

13.1.1.8. Make a Long-Term Commitment

Related to the fact that there is no "magic cure" in these areas, recovery is usually a long-term process. This requires some counseling and therapeutic relations lasting for at least a year.

13.1.1.9. Use All Available Resources

The patient's substance-abuse problem does not occur in a vacuum. Part of the therapeutic effort should be directed at encouraging the family and, if appropriate, the employer to increase his/her level of understanding of the problem; to be available to help you whenever necessary; to make realistic plans for themselves as they relate to the patient; and, in specific instances, to function as "ancillary therapists," helping to carry out your treatment efforts in the home or job setting.

13.1.1.10. When Appropriate, Notify All Involved Physicians and Pharmacists

When dealing with a substance misuser who is obtaining drugs from physicians or pharmacists, it is my *bias* to make all possible efforts to cut off the patient's supply. This must be done with tact, understanding, and empathy for the ego of the prescribing physician or dispensing pharmacist involved and with the patient's permission, to avoid infringing on his legal rights.

13.1.1.11. Do Not Take Final Responsibility on the Patient's Actions

Although I do everything within my power to help, in the final analysis the decision to achieve and maintain abstinence is the patient's responsibility. If I do not follow this rule and the patient stops only to please me, he'll soon find an excuse to get angry with me and return to alcohol and/or drugs.

13.1.2. A "General" Substance-Abuse Treatment Program

Recognizing that there are patients in need, that money is available for care, and that there is a great deal of pressure to "do something now," it is possible to establish a rehabilitation program that will *probably* do the most good with the least harm. I emphasize the probable nature of my recommendations, as adequately controlled investigations have rarely been carried out in testing even the most basic assumptions in rehabilitation. The *usual* rehabilitation program would[1]:

1. Keep the inpatient phase short (usually less than 2–3 weeks), as longer inpatient care has not been demonstrated to be more effective than short-term care for the average patient.

2. Avoid using most medications in the treatment of substance misuse after withdrawal is completed. Possible exceptions are disulfiram (Antabuse) for alcoholism and methadone for opiate abuse.

3. Use group more than individual counseling, as the former costs less and is probably equally effective.

4. Use self-help groups such as Alcoholics Anonymous, as they can be quite helpful while costing little. They offer the patient a model that may be important in achieving and maintaining recovery.

5. Recognize that there is no evidence that specialized and expensive forms of psychotherapy (e.g., gestalt or transactional analysis) are any more effective than general "day-to-day" life counseling for the substance misuser.

6. Maintain continued contact with the patient for at least a year after formal rehabilitation has ended.

7. Use nondegreed (paraprofessional) counseling staff supervised by staff with more formal training in counselling, as there is little evidence that treatment must be carried out by individuals with advanced degrees in order to be successful.

13.2. A SPECIAL CASE: ALCOHOLISM

Because alcoholism is the most common substance of abuse, I will use it as a prototype for my discussion of all other types of rehabilitation. A general outline of this approach is given in Figure 13.1.

13.2.1. General Treatment Philosophy

Alcoholism is characterized by a fluctuating course, and the alcoholic has approximately a 10–30% chance of reaching "spontaneous remission."[2] It is my *bias* that, before interfering in a person's life, the therapist must understand the expected course of the disorder and have a method for choosing among the various treatments. It is best to avoid dramatic fads, which, historically, result in a number of miraculous "cures" and too often are discovered to be doing harm. I evaluate treatment efforts and new approaches reported in the literature with special care, requiring

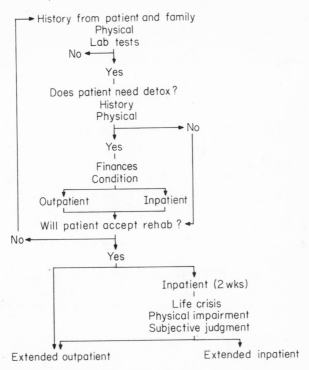

Is the problem alcohol related ?

Figure 13.1. Discussions in alcoholism treatment. From Schuckit, M. A. Treatment of alcoholism in office and outpatient settings. In J. H. Mendelson & N. K. Mello (Eds.), *Diagnosis and Treatment of Alcoholism*. New York: McGraw-Hill, copyright © 1979. Reprinted with permission of the McGraw-Hill Book Company.

evidence of efficacy and some measure of a justifiable cost–benefit ratio before I am impressed.

13.2.2. Confrontation of the Alcoholic

If an individual might have serious alcohol problems, gather as much information as possible from a spouse or other relevant resource person; then share your concerns with the patient, using his presenting complaint as an entrée into alcohol problems. Teach him about the future difficulties that he can expect unless he stops drinking, and tell him that it appears that he has reached a point in life where he can no longer tolerate alcohol.[5] I think that it is not necessary to use the term *alcoholism* at this stage, but rather, in the initial confrontation, alcohol-related life problems can be the focus.

For instance, for a person coming for a "checkup" because he doesn't "feel well," share the results of your evaluations or laboratory tests and physical findings, and, when relevant, describe the ways in which alcohol has probably caused much of the problem. Next, discuss the probable future course of alcohol problems and explore possible avenues for treatment. If he accepts help, determine if detox is required and either begin counseling or refer him to Alcoholics Anonymous or to an appropriate inpatient or outpatient facility.

13.2.3. Enhancing Motivation

It is important to establish and increase the patient's recognition of and desire to stop alcohol-related problems.[6] The enhancement of motivation is complex and centers on the attitudes of the therapist, the ability of treatment to meet the patient's unique needs, and the attitudes of important individuals, such as his family, friends, and employer. The therapist can do much to help improve motivation through working with all available resources.[7]

For those patients who refuse care, keep the door open and encourage the patient and his family to remain in contact, but be careful not to push so hard that the patient either allows you to take over totally or becomes put off by an overbearing attitude.

13.2.4. Treatment Programs

13.2.4.1. Inpatient Treatment

Selection of an inpatient or an outpatient treatment mode is based on the preferences of the patient or client and his family, financial considerations, and your prior experiences. Although there are no absolute indications for hospitalization after detoxification, patients with serious medical or emotional problems, or those who face severe crises, will probably function best in a structured environment. Also most health care deliverers feel that a short "time out" from life stresses is an important part of treating the average alcoholic.

There are no data to support hospitalization of more than two or three weeks for the *average* patient.[8,9,15,16] Of course, common sense dictates that individuals with severe medical problems or persistent organic brain syndromes or those with very unstable life situations might require longer care. It is important, however, to recognize the potential dangers associated with inpatient care which include exposure to risks of treatment-center–acquired infections, physical or emotional harm by patients or staff, loss of income or loss of job, embarrassment among peers, and family dissolution through separation at a time of crisis. In addition, the patient is treated in an artificial environment where lessons learned may not readily generalize to everyday living.[8] Although inpatient care is a potentially important part of the rehabilitation spectrum, final decisions should depend upon a calculated balance between the negative and positive aspects of any program.

13.2.4.1.1. The Facility

Good alcoholic detoxification and rehabilitation can be carried out in an established alcoholic program or on a general medical ward,[10] the latter being especially important when you are dealing with a patient with serious medical problems or one who refuses care from anyone other than his primary physician. In such instances, the primary treatment is medical, but the counselor can work with the treatment staff to carry out adequate detoxification, if needed, and to enhance the patient's receptiveness to rehabilitation.

In a similar manner, patients with primary affective disorder and secondary alcoholism (see Section 3.1.2.3.) are best treated by a psychiatrist. If these patients have active suicidal ideation, care should be given in a psychiatric facility where suicide precautions can be taken. After detoxification, active pharmacologic treatment of the affective disorder can be carried out. For patients presenting with depressions who have no histories of manias, this usually entails the same treatment given any patient with unipolar affective disorders, usually tricyclic antidepressants, while patients who have both manias and depressions respond best to lithium. The reader is referred to some excellent reviews of the proper use of medications in primary affective disorder.[4,11,12] The data to date, however, do *not* justify the routine use of antidepressants or lithium in the average primary alcoholic.

The very rare alcoholic with process schizophrenia[4] will require relatively high doses of antipsychotic medications such as chlorpromazine (Thorazine). The clinician must take special care not to misdiagnose alcoholic psychosis as schizophrenia (see Section 4.2.4.)

13.2.4.1.2. The Daily Schedule

Rehabilitation centers on offering good education, counseling for the patient *and his family*, and a long-term commitment to help with life adjustment. The usual inpatient schedule offers daily educational lectures and/or films, along with daily counseling and "rap" sessions, and, in some centers, behavior modification therapy. Most programs favor a busy daily schedule.

13.2.4.1.3. Counseling or Psychotherapy

The patient usually meets with a counselor in a group setting daily to clarify life adjustment issues and set the stage for outpatient follow-up visits. The family should be included in some sessions to help them deal with the life problems and to increase their level of understanding of alcoholism.

Therapy generally centers on the "here and now" of the patient's life, giving him a chance to discuss his adjustment to a life without alcohol and to the stresses of job, friends, and family, with a focus on the reactions of those around him and on how to handle situations in which he is most likely to return to drinking. In addition, lecture/discussion sessions can emphasize the dangers of alcohol and help the patient understand the course and effects of his disease. Along with other forms of therapy, patients should be encouraged to take part in Alcoholics Anonymous (AA).

Comparisons of group and individual psychotherapy for alcoholism reveal that group therapy is as effective.[13] Some authors may feel that group therapy has specific *advantages*, such as allowing the patient to share his feelings with a number of other people and teaching him social skills,[14] however, there is little hard evidence to back this up. The group session is an excellent place to begin an interdisciplinary approach,[15] with the physician or psychologist being used primarily to supervise other therapists.

13.2.4.1.4. Behavioral Approaches

Many alcoholism treatment programs utilize some form of behavioral approach in dealing with their patients. This may include the offering of supports like biofeedback, which teach the patient how to relax and handle stress. Another behaviorally oriented intervention, assertiveness training, is based on the premise that in the midst of their alcoholism (or perhaps reflecting some original problem existing before the alcoholism began) most patients do not learn how to express their desires and frustrations.[16] The training sessions usually involve education about recognizing situations in which resentment occurs and practicing a variety of methods for handling them.

Some programs utilize behavioral approaches as a core program in the treatment of alcoholism, with the behavioral modification procedures usually added to the regular education and counselling as previously described. Most often, this involves attempts to "teach" the patient not to drink through coupling the sight, scent, or taste of alcohol with an unpleasant event, such as vomiting or receiving a mild electric shock to the skin.[17-19] Chemical aversion treatments, aimed at inducing vomiting in the presence of alcohol, usually utilize such substances as emetine or apomorphine and are generally felt to be more effective than electrical aversion. These treatments are usually offered in hospitals that have special experience with them, and controlled studies indicate the approach is as effective as any other in dealing with alcoholism. Although it is possible that a specific type of patient responds preferentially to behavioral interventions, there are no data to help us choose those individuals.

One modification of the electrical aversion treatment attempts to teach alcoholics the mechanisms to help them drink in a moderate, controlled manner. This approach may have some potential, but, at present, the data are far too tenuous to justify its use in any clinical setting. Use outside of the experimental laboratory must await clear demonstration that the assets of such a treatment outweigh the liabilities.

13.2.4.1.5. Medications

1. It is important to remember that any treatment, especially medications, when given as part of uncontrolled clinical evaluations can appear effective; but, in reality, it may be no better than placebo.[1,20] Therefore, with the possible exception of disulfiram (Antabuse) and vitamins, I tend to use *no* medications in treating the detoxified alcoholic.

2. Sleeping pills and antianxiety drugs, even though the patient may demand them, have no place in alcoholic *rehabilitation* (after withdrawal is completed). These drugs have dangers of addiction, adverse reactions with other depressant drugs such as alcohol, and, for most hypnotics, the potential for overdosage.

I use a special approach in dealing with complaints of insomnia and/or anxiety in the alcoholic. First, I let them know that I understand the intensity of their discomfort and that I will try to help them. Secondly, I tell them that many of their problems are a physiological response to the long-term self-administration of a brain depressing drug and that these physical changes will persist for up to six months, although at decreasing intensity. Thirdly, I emphasize that sleeping pills or antianxiety drugs might help them for a week or two but will then make their problems worse, and that we will inevitably have to face the day where their body must adjust to living without CNS depressing medications.

To help them deal with their sleep difficulties, I prescribe a regimen of going to bed at the same time every night (reading or watching television, if needed) and awakening at the same time every morning, even if they have had only 15 minutes of good sleep. This is coupled with a rule against caffeinated beverages after noon, and no naps during the day—all of which combine to force the patient's sleep cycle into a more normal pattern after several days. Problems with anxiety are handled with similar types of explanation and a search, carried out jointly with the patient, to find nonmedicinal avenues for release of tension. Possibilities range from church work, to developing a hobby, to learning to play a musical instrument, to yoga, to physical exercise, etc.

3. Disulfiram (Antabuse) is a promising drug for the treatment of the alcoholic, but this substance has dangers and cannot be given to patients with serious medical disorders.[21] Although Antabuse does not decrease the "drive" to drink, knowledge of a possible severe physical reaction following drinking for patients on Antabuse is associated with an improved recovery rate.[8,22] The drug is given orally, usually at a daily dose of 250 mg, over an extended period of time, perhaps up to a year. Investigators are currently working on the development of a long-lasting implant, but present methods have not been successful in maintaining adequate blood levels of the drug.[23] Antabuse is *not* an effective agent for aversive conditioning, because the time lag between ingestion of alcohol and the reaction is often delayed up to 30 minutes, and the intensity of the reaction is unpredictable.

13.2.4.2. Outpatient Programs

Although it is assumed that you will be offering alcoholic rehabilitation, there are also a variety of outpatient programs available for referral. These range from private care to clinics to the outpatient extensions of inpatient programs. One valuable information resource is the National Council on Alcoholism (NCA) (usually listed in the telephone book), which in most urban areas will act as a referral source. Many communities also have state- or county-operated evaluation centers that can be reached through government-run health services.

In addition, many alcoholics have life crisis problems or vocational rehabilitation needs. Referral to a social service agency, a visiting nurses association, or state vocational rehabilitation offices can be most helpful.

The same general approach applies both to patients who have never been hospitalized and to those beginning an aftercare program. The patient is counseled about day-to-day life adjustments and helped to deal with crisis situations. After a period of time, life adjustment tends to stabilize, and the patient incorporates enough of the messages being presented by the counselor to stop formal treatment.

Usually, counseling is begun at a frequency of one a week, but then it is slowly decreased so that after a year the patient is seen about once a month. If problems with drinking or life adjustment occur, the frequency of meeting can be increased to meet the acute need.

For the *secondary alcoholic* (see Section 3.1.2.3.) who does not require inpatient care, referral to a mental health specialist should be considered. If the diagnosis is primary affective disorder, but the patient is *not* felt to be severely incapacitated or suicidal (in which case he should be hospitalized), outpatient treatment with antidepressants is possible. In such instances, the patient should be referred either to a psychiatric clinic or to a psychiatrist for evaluation.

In delivering care to the alcoholic with a primary *antisocial personality*, it is necessary to recognize the high rates of concomitant drug abuse and the elevated risk for commission of serious crimes in these individuals.[24] There is no highly effective treatment known, but some authors favor heavily structured group sessions following a therapeutic community model.[25] Outpatient referral to an experienced health specialist is advisable, as there is no evidence that inpatient care is routinely justified.

Some individuals are not ready to return to their day-to-day life after inpatient treatment. If the problem is either chronic medical or psychiatric impairment, a nursing home or halfway house should be considered. For those with more serious problems, a nursing home is probably required, but, whenever possible, this should be integrated with continued outpatient treatment and AA.

These nursing or halfway settings usually offer continued group meetings, supervision of medications, and help in dealing with emotional problems and crises. As is true with any of the modes of treatment, it is important that the clinician carefully evaluate each individual program before actual referral.[26]

13.2.4.3. The Role of Alcoholics Anonymous

Alcoholics Anonymous is an excellent resource for treatment.[27] This group, composed of individuals who are themselves recovering alcoholics (many of whom have been "dry" for years), establishes a milieu where help is available 24 hours a day, seven days a week.[5] At meetings, members share their own recovery experiences, demonstrating to the patient that he is not alone and that a better lifestyle is possible. AA also offers help in the form of groups that discuss the special problems of children of alcoholics (Alateen) and of spouses (Alanon). Each AA group has its own personality, and the patient might experiment with different groups before choosing the one in which he is most comfortable.

AA can be used as a referral resource where no other outpatient service is either available or acceptable to the patient. It can also be utilized as an adjunct to outpatient or inpatient treatment efforts.

13.2.4.4. An Overview

In summary, the majority of time in alcoholic rehabilitation is spent in outpatient settings. Therapy involves a commonsense approach to group counseling, a long-term follow-up, working with the patient and family together, and avoiding most medications. There is no place in alcoholic rehabilitation for antianxiety drugs or hypnotics. Disulfiram has dangers and cannot be utilized for all patients, but it is a useful adjunct for medically healthy individuals who willingly take it.

13.3. A SPECIAL CASE: OPIATES

The opiate abuser differs from the alcoholic in that the former tends to be younger and to have more antisocial problems, comes from different referral sources (e.g., jail or probation), and more often abuses ancillary drugs. The high level of crime associated with the illicit use of opiates has necessitated the development of a "maintenance" program that is purported to result in lowered levels of antisocial activities[28] but that does not deal with the basic addiction. Even with these differences, however, the same general rules for rehabilitation apply to the opiate abuser and the alcoholic. These "basics" include: detoxification, the need to reach out to the family, the need to carefully evaluate efforts, establishing patient goals and a program of counselling giving drug education, and making a long-term commitment to the patient. I will, therefore, concentrate on specific aspects of rehabilitation of the opiate abuser that have not already been covered.

Various additional forms of treatment include:

13.3.1. Methadone and Methadyl Acetate Maintenance

Methadone and methadyl acetate maintenance can be given only in licensed clinics established to ensure adequate care and to minimize the flow of methadone into illegal channels.[29]

13.3.1.1. Goals

Methadone does not "cure" opiate addiction. The program substitutes legal access to a longer-acting drug (e.g., methadone) for the addiction to a shorter-acting drug such as heroin. Methadone maintenance is used to help the addict develop a lifestyle free of street drugs in order to improve functioning within the family and job, to decrease police problems, and to enhance health status.[28]

Methadone should be given only as part of a holistic patient approach, incorporating all the other aspects of rehabilitation thus far described.[30] In this therapy, it is hoped that, if the addict receives a drug legally (orally, to avoid the "rush" felt with IV drugs), at little or no cost, he will not return to the costs and problems inherent in street drugs. At the same time, methadone is felt to decrease drug craving and to (at least partially) block the "high" experienced with heroin.

13.3.1.2. Treatment Program

Methadone is a long-acting opiate that shares almost all the physiological properties of heroin including addiction, sedation, respiratory depression, and effects on heart and muscle. The addict who has been carefully screened to rule out prior psychiatric disorders may be maintained on a relatively *low* (30–40 mg a day) or higher dose (100–120 mg a day) methadone schedule, the former giving less side effects but not the same degree of hypothetical "blockade" against the effects of heroin.[30,31] The drug is administered in an oral liquid given once a day at the program center, with weekend doses taken by the patient at home. An approach similar to methadone maintenance utilizes a longer-acting methadone congener, methadyl acetate.[34] The dosage is usually 20–30 mg given three times a week in the beginning, then increased to 80 mg, if necessary. Available evidence indicates that the results are similar to those with methadone.

After the period of maintenance (usually six months to a year, or longer), the clinician should work closely with the patient to regulate the rate of drug decrease.[32] Most studies suggest that the dose be lowered as slowly as 3% a week.[33]

Methadone-type drugs have been taken by some individuals for over 10 years and are *felt* by clinicians to be relatively safe and effective.[34,35] However, the dangers associated with these drugs include the relatively benign side effect of constipation (seen in 17%),[36] the danger of addicting the fetus when the drug is given during pregnancy, a potentially serious depression,[37] and the possibility that the drug will find its way into illegal channels. Another special problem (seen in as high as one-quarter of methadone maintenance patients) is abuse of alcohol, especially for those individuals who abused alcohol before using the opiates, or who took alcohol concomitantly with their opiate abuse.[38]

13.3.2. Opiate Antagonists

These drugs occupy opiate receptors in the brain and block the effects of heroin and other opiates.[30] Concomitant administration of the antagonist with heroin stops the development of physical dependence but does not block the drug hunger (psychological dependence).[36]

13.3.2.1. Goals

Use of antagonists is not limited to rehabilitation. They help treat the opiate toxic reactions and can be used to test addicts who say they are drug-free (the antagonist will precipitate withdrawal if opiates have been abused).[30] In rehabilitation, however, these drugs are administered over an extended period so that the patient cannot develop a dependence on opiates.

13.3.2.2. Specific Antagonists

There are a variety of opiate antagonists, most of which are themselves addicting. These drugs include the following:

1. *Cyclazocine* is an antagonist administered orally in doses of 4–6 mg and has a length of action of approximately 24 hours. However, this drug has sedative side effects and produces physical dependence because of its strong agonistic properties[30] and thus has not been widely used.[39]

2. *Naloxone* (Narcan) is an excellent narcotic antagonist that has no known agonistic properties. Unfortunately, it is not well absorbed orally, and its actions last no more than two to three hours.[39]

3. *Nalorphene* (Nalline) is primarily used to test addiction to opiates. It is administered in a dark room; if the individual is addicted, pupillary dilatation is seen within 15 minutes to half an hour, whereas if no addiction is present, pupillary constriction is seen. If no reaction at all is noted, 5 mg and then 7 mg can be given at half-hour intervals.[39] This drug is not usually used as a rehabilitative agent.

4. *Noroxymorphone* (Naltrexone) is a widely used narcotic antagonist that can be given orally, has a length of action of approximately 24 hours, and has few side effects.[40,41] It is usually given three mornings a week, with 100 mg on Monday and Wednesday and 150 mg on Friday. Some programs use between 40 and 200 mg a day, beginning with doses of 10–100 mg per day and increasing slowly. Considering its length of action, clients should receive a test dose (0.8 mg) of naloxone to be sure that they are not dependent before regular use is begun.

13.3.3. Other Drugs Used in Treatment

Any disorder with a natural history that includes periods of improvement with a relatively high rate of spontaneous remission runs the danger of having a variety of touted, but ineffective treatments. Uncontrolled experiments have extolled such misleading cures as carbon dioxide inhalation and LSD.[33] I will mention only a few of the more promising approaches here.

1. *Propoxyphene* (Darvon) has cross-tolerance with other opiates and has been used as a method of detoxification from opiate addiction. Be-

cause of the belief that this drug has less appeal on the street and lower side effects than some other medications, short-term "maintenance" with this medication (approximately three weeks) has been used but has not been shown to be uniquely effective.[42]

2. *Propranolol* (Inderal) in doses of from 5 to 120 mg per day has been administered to block the immediate "rush" or "high" seen with heroin.[43] Uncontrolled studies indicate a decrease in drug craving, but better-controlled evaluations are necessary before this drug is used in general settings.

3. *Clonidine* in doses 5 μg/kg is a promising *experimental drug* for treating opiate withdrawal.[44] The drug appears to decrease markedly abstinence symptoms through an inhibition of nonadrenaline activity in the alpha–2 receptors, especially in the locus coeruleus area of the brain.

4. *Heroin* itself has been administered as part of a maintenance program.[45] The rationale here is similar to that offered for methadone; that is, it is used to decrease the necessity for getting the drug on the street and to cut down on the medical complications from adulterated drugs and contaminated needles. It has been used primarily in Britain, where the magnitude of opiate problems is very small compared to those of the United States (it is estimated that there were only 500 addicts in Britain when heroin maintenance was begun). After it became legal to prescribe heroin, the number of addicts doubled, necessitating the establishment of clinics similar to methadone maintenance programs. It is now uncommon to find a clinic in Britain that prescribes heroin and only heroin, as most are turning toward methadone maintenance.

13.3.4. Drug-Free Programs

Most inpatient treatment models offered to the opiate abuser utilize modifications of the therapeutic community, as first proposed by Jones.[46] This is an exception to the general rule of short-term inpatient rehabilitation, as it lasts up to a year while the addict is taken out of the street culture and given a new identity within the group. In this structure, group members, including ex-addict leaders, constantly confront each behavior in an attempt to help participants gain insight and find a new and more successful lifestyle for coping with problems. Most large communities in the United States have programs run on the Synanon or Day Top models.[36] Unfortunately, very little controlled evaluation has been carried out regarding this approach.

13.3.5. The Medical Abuser

The middle-class individual primarily abusing prescription opiates may be more similar to the alcoholic in general life outlook and history than to the street abusers of opiates. There is little good information on the best rehabilitation mode for this population, and the final program should be tailored to the specific patient, perhaps using the same approach applied to alcohol.

13.4. A SPECIAL CASE: HALLUCINOGENS, STIMULANTS, DEPRESSANTS, AND MULTIDRUG MISUSE

It is rarely necessary to establish specific rehabilitation efforts for individuals who are "casual" users of marijuana or hallucinogens. However, serious consequences can occur when hallucinogens are used regularly or in high doses and when stimulants or depressants are regularly ingested. Because there is a high level of correlation between heavy misuse of any one of these substances and the use of multiple drugs, I will present a discussion that is fitted primarily to the multidrug misuser but that can also be applied to those individuals involved with only one type of substance.

After establishing the diagnosis, carrying out detoxification, if necessary, and ruling out the possibility of any major preexisting psychiatric disorder, the next step is to determine questions:

1. Is the individual primarily abusing street drugs or taking medications prescribed by a physician?
2. Is there a primary or preferred drug of misuse?
3. Under what circumstances does the individual misuse multiple drugs?
4. Is the client a member of a street subculture of drug users or a middle-class, blue-collar or white-collar working individual?

In a program dealing primarily with street users, the more middle-class individual may be referred to a more appropriate program. This type of flexibility is of great importance in giving the patient an adequate and comfortable milieu. The actual treatment protocol chosen will resemble either the efforts described for alcoholism or, for the person more heavily involved in the street culture, those described under drug-free program for opiates. Each individual client's needs, of course, must be considered in designing patient rehabilitation plans.

REFERENCES

1. Schuckit, M. A., & Cahalan, D. Evaluation of alcoholism treatment programs. In W. J. Filstead, J. J. Rossi, & M. Keller (Eds.), *Alcohol and Alcohol Problems: New Thinking and New Directions.* Cambridge, Mass.: Ballinger, 1976.

2. Smart, R. G. Spontaneous recovery in alcoholics. *Drug and Alcohol Dependence.* 1:277–285, 1976.

3. Vaillant, G. E. A 20-year follow-up of New York narcotic addicts. *Archives of General Psychiatry.* 29:237–241, 1973.

4. Woodruff, R. A., Jr., Goodwin, D. W., & Guze, S. B. *Psychiatric Diagnosis.* New York: Oxford University Press, 1974.

5. Schuckit, M. A. Treatment of alcoholism in office and outpatient settings. In J. H. Mendelson & N. K. Mello (Eds.), *Diagnosis and Treatment of Alcoholism,* Chapter 6. New York. McGraw-Hill, 1979.

6. Rossi, J. J., & Filstead, M. J. Treating the treatment issues. In M. J. Filstead, J. J. Rossi, & M. Keller (Eds.), *Alcohol and Alcohol Problems.* Cambridge, Mass.: Ballinger, 1976, pp. 193–228.

7. Fox, R. Treatment of the problem drinker by private practitioners. In P. G. Bourne & R. Fox (Eds.), *Alcoholism, Progress in Research and Treatment.* New York: Academic Press, 1973, pp. 227–244.

8. Schuckit, M. A. Inpatient and residential approaches to the treatment of alcoholism. In J. H. Mendelson & N. K. Mello (Eds.), *Diagnosis and Treatment of Alcoholism.* Chapter 7. New York: McGraw-Hill, 1979.

9. Edwards, G., Orford, J., Egert, S., *et al.* Alcoholism: A controlled trial of "treatment" and "advice." *Journal of Studies on Alcohol.* 38:1004–1031, 1977.

10. West, J. W. The general hospital as a primary setting for the treatment of alcoholism. Presented at the National Council on Alcoholism Seventh Annual Conference, Washington, D.C., May 1976.

11. Hollister, L. E. *Clinical Use of Psychotherapeutic Drugs.* Springfield, Ill.: Charles C Thomas, 1975, pp. 56–110.

12. Baldessarini, R. J. *Chemotherapy in Psychiatry.* Cambridge, Mass.: Harvard University Press, 1977, pp. 57–125.

13. Emrick, C. D. A review of psychologically oriented treatment of alcoholism. II. *Journal of Studies on Alcohol.* 36:88–108, 1975.

14. Forrest, G. G. *The Diagnosis and Treatment of Alcoholism.* Springfield, Ill.: Charles C Thomas, 1975.

15. Brown, S., & Yalom, I. D. Interactional group therapy with alcoholics. *Journal of Studies on Alcohol.* 38:426–456, 1977.

16. Briddell, D. W., & Nathan, P. E. Behavior assessment and modification with alcoholics: Current status and future trends. In M. Hersen, R. Eisler, & P. Miller (Eds.), *Progress in Behavior Modification,* Vol. II. New York: Academic Press, 1976.

17. Miller, P. M., & Barlow, D. H. Behavioral approaches to the treatment of alcoholism. *Journal of Nervous and Mental Disease.* 157:10–20, 1973.

18. Glover, J. H., & McCue, P. A. Electrical aversion therapy with alcoholics. *British Journal of Psychiatry.* 130:279–286, 1977.

19. Nathan, P. E., & Lisman, S. A. Behavioral and motivational patterns of chronic alcoholics. In R. E. Tartar & A. A. Sugarman (Eds.), *Alcoholism: Interdisciplinary Approaches to an Enduring Problem.* Reading, Mass.: Addison-Wesley, 1976.

20. Goodwin, D. W., & Reinhard, J. Disulfiram-like effects of trichomonacidal drugs: A review and double blind study. *Quarterly Journal of Studies on Alcohol.* 33:734–740, 1972.

21. Kitson, T. M. The disulfiram–ethanol reaction. *Journal of Studies on Alcohol.* 38:96–113, 1977.

22. Wilson, A., Davidson, W. J., & White, J. Disulfiram implantation: Placebo, psychological deterrent, and pharmacological detterent effects. *British Journal of Psychiatry.* 129:277–280, 1976.
23. Wilson, A. Disulfiram implantation in alcoholism treatment. A review. *Journal of Studies on Alcohol.* 36:555–565, 1975.
24. Schuckit, M. A. Alcoholism and sociopathy: Diagnostic confusion. *Quarterly Journal of Studies on Alcohol.* 34:157–164, 1973.
25. Whiteley, J. S. The response of psychopaths to a therapeutic community. *British Journal of Psychiatry.* 116:517–529, 1970.
26. Baker, T. B., Sobell, M. B., & Sobell, L. C. Halfway houses for alcoholics: A review analysis and comparison with other halfway house facilities. *International Journal of Social Psychiatry.* 22:1–7, 1976.
27. O. G. Alcoholics Anonymous. *Journal of the American Medical Association.* 236:1505–1506, 1976.
28. Goldstein, A. Heroin addiction. Sequential treatment employing pharmacologic supports. *Archives of General Psychiatry.* 33:353–358, 1976.
29. Stephens, R. C., & Weppner, R. S. Legal and illegal use of methadone: One year later. *American Journal of Psychiatry.* 130(12):1391–1394, 1973.
30. Jaffe, J. H. Drug addiction and drug abuse. In L. S. Goodman & A. Gilman (Eds.), *The Pharmacological Basis of Therapeutics.* New York: Macmillan, 1975, pp. 293–324.
31. Goldstein, A., Hansteen, R. W., & Horns, M. H. Control of methadone dosage by patients. *Journal of the American Medical Association.* 234(7):734–737, 1975.
32. Razani, J., Chilholm, D., Glasser, M., *et al.* Self-regulated methadone detoxification of heroin addicts. An improved technique in an inpatient setting. *Archives of General Psychiatry.* 32:909–911, 1975.
33. Senay, E. C., Dorus, W., Goldberg, F., *et al.* Withdrawal from methadone maintenance. Rate of withdrawal and expectation. *Archives of General Psychiatry.* 34:361–368, 1977.
34. Ling, W., Charuvastra, V. C., Kaim, S. C., *et al.* Methadyl acetate and methadone as maintenance treatments for heroin addicts. *Archives of General Psychiatry.* 33:709–720, 1976.
35. Newman, R. G. Methadone maintenance: It ain't what it used to be. *British Journal of Addictions.* 71:183–186, 1976.
36. Stimmel, B. *Heroin Dependency: Medical, Economic, and Social Aspects.* New York: Stratton Intercontinental Medical Book Corporation, 1975.
37. Weissman, M. M., Slobetz, F., Prusoff, B., *et al.* Clinical depression among narcotic addicts maintained on methadone in the community. *American Journal of Psychiatry.* 133(12):1434–1438, 1976.
38. Green, J., & Jaffe, J. H. Alcohol and opiate dependence. A review. *Journal of Studies on Alcohol.* 38(7):1274–1293, 1977.
39. Shapira, J. *Drug Abuse: A Guide for the Clinician.* New York: American Elsevier, 1975, pp. 319–333.
40. Brahan, L. S., Capone, T., Wiechert, V., *et al.* Naltrexone and cyclazocine. A controlled treatment study. *Archives of General Psychiatry.* 34:1181–1184, 1977.
41. Volavka, J., Resnick, R. B., Kestenbaum, R. S., *et al.* Short-term effects of naltrexone in 155 heroin ex-addicts. *Biological Psychiatry.* 11(6):679–685, 1976.

42. Tennant, F. S., Jr. Propoxyphene napsylate for heroin addiction. *Journal of the American Medical Association*. 226(8):1012, 1973.

43. Grosz, H. J. Propranolol in the treatment of heroin dependence. In H. Bostrum (Ed.), *Skandia International Symposia: Drug Dependence, Treatment and Treatment Evaluation*. Stockholm: Bastrum, 1974.

44. Gold, M. S., Redmond, D. E., & Kleber H. D. Noradrenergic hyperactivity in opiate withdrawal. *American Journal of Psychiatry*. 136:100–101, 1979.

45. Lidz, C. W., Lewis, S. H., Crane, L. E., *et al*. Heroin maintenance and heroin control. *International Journal of Addictions*. 10(1):35–52, 1975.

46. Romond, A. M., Forrest, C. K., & Kleber, H. D. Follow-up of participants in a drug dependence therapeutic community. *Archives of General Psychiatry*. 32:369–374, 1975.

Index